LIPPINCOTT'S PHOTO ATLAS OF MEDICATION ADMINISTRATION

Second Edition

9   8   7   6

ISBN 0-7817-6318-5

Care has been taken to confirm the accuracy of the information presented and to describe generally accepted practices. However, the author, editors, and publisher are not responsible for errors or omissions or for any consequences from application of the information in this book and make no warranty, express or implied, with respect to the content of the publication.

The author, editors, and publisher have exerted every effort to ensure that drug selection and dosage set forth in this text are in accordance with the current recommendations and practice at the time of publication. However, in view of ongoing research, changes in government regulations, and the constant flow of information relating to drug therapy and drug reactions, the reader is urged to check the package insert for each drug for any change in indications and dosage and for added warnings and precautions. This is particularly important when the recommended agent is a new or infrequently employed drug.

Some drugs and medical devices presented in this publication have Food and Drug Administration (FDA) clearance for limited use in restricted research settings. It is the responsibility of the health care provider to ascertain the FDA status of each drug or device planned for use in his or her clinical practice.

LWW.com

LIPPINCOTT'S PHOTO ATLAS OF MEDICATION ADMINISTRATION

Second Edition

Pamela Evans-Smith, MSN, FNP

Clinical Nursing Instructor

University of Missouri

Columbia, Missouri

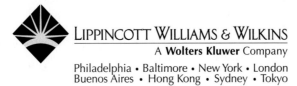

LIPPINCOTT WILLIAMS & WILKINS
A **Wolters Kluwer** Company

Philadelphia • Baltimore • New York • London
Buenos Aires • Hong Kong • Sydney • Tokyo

Medication administration is a basic nursing function that involves skillful technique and consideration of the patient's development and safety. The nurse administering medications needs a knowledge base about drugs, including drug names, preparations, classifications, adverse effects, and physiologic factors that affect drug action.

The nursing process can be applied to the fundamental nursing skill of medication administration. Assessment includes a comprehensive medication history as well as ongoing assessments of the patient's response during and after drug therapy. Nursing diagnoses are developed from the assessment data. Patient-centered outcomes are evaluated after implementation of the plan of care, tailored to the patient's needs.

This chapter will cover skills that the nurse needs to safely administer medications via several routes. Please look over the summary boxes in the beginning of this chapter for a quick review of critical knowledge to assist you in understanding the skills related to medication administration.

BOX 1 Five Rights of Administration

To prevent medication errors, always check the Five Rights of Medication Administration:

1. Right patient
2. Right medication
3. Right dosage
4. Right route
5. Right time

BOX 2 Clarifying Orders

Another way to prevent medication errors is always to clarify a medication order that is:

- Illegible
- Incomplete
- Incorrect route or dosage
- Not expected for patient's current diagnosis

BOX 3 Know Your Medications

Before administering any unfamiliar medications, know the following:

- Mode of action and purpose of medication (making sure that this medication is appropriate for the patient's diagnosis)
- Side effects of and contraindications for medication
- Antagonist of medication
- Safe dosage range for medication
- Interactions with other medications
- Precautions to take prior to administration
- Proper administration technique

BOX 4 Needle/Syringe Selection Technique

- When looking at a needle package, the first number is the gauge or diameter of the needle (eg, 18, 20) and the second number is the length in inches (eg 1, 1½).
- As the gauge number becomes larger, the size of the needle becomes smaller: for instance, a 24-gauge needle is smaller than an 18-gauge needle.
- When giving an injection, the viscosity of the medication directs the choice of gauge (diameter). A thicker medication such as a hormone is given through a bigger needle, such as a 20 gauge. A thinner-consistency medication, such as morphine, is given through a smaller needle, such as a 24 gauge.
- The length of the needle is directed by the size of the patient, the selected insertion site, and the tissue you are trying to reach. An intramuscular injection in an emaciated person would require a shorter needle than the same injection in an obese patient.
- Generally, a 1½" needle is sufficient for an intramuscular injection in an adult and a 1" needle is sufficient for a

child. A ⁵⁄₁₆" to 1" needle is generally used for subcutaneous injections.
- The size of the syringe is directed by the amount of medication to be given. If the amount is less than 1 mL, use a 1-mL syringe to administer the medication. In a 1-mL syringe, the amount of medication may be rounded to the 100th decimal place. In syringes larger than 1 mL, the amount is rounded to the 10th decimal place. If the amount of medication to be administered is less than 3 mL, use a 3-mL syringe. If the amount of medication is equal to the size of the syringe (eg, 1 mL and using a 1-mL syringe), you may go up to the next size syringe to prevent awkward movements when deploying the plunger.
- When administering insulin, the size of syringe and strength of insulin should coincide. U50 insulin should be administered with a syringe calibrated for U50 insulin to prevent medication errors.

continues

BOX 4 **Needle/Syringe Selection Technique** (*continued*)

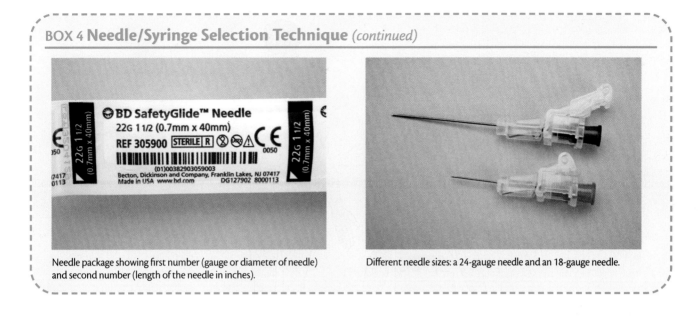

Needle package showing first number (gauge or diameter of needle) and second number (length of the needle in inches).

Different needle sizes: a 24-gauge needle and an 18-gauge needle.

BOX 5 **Subcutaneous Injections**

- Subcutaneous injections should contain no more than 1 mL of fluid in one insertion site.
- The normal angle for insertion for a subcutaneous injection is 45 to 90 degrees. This angle depends on the length of the needle and the amount of adipose tissue the patient has. An emaciated patient would probably require a 45-degree angle of insertion, while an obese patient may require a 90-degree angle.
- Subcutaneous injection sites include:
  - Outer aspect of upper arm
  - Abdomen
  - Anterior aspects of thigh
  - Upper back
  - Upper ventral or dorsogluteal area
- Insertion site selection depends on patient's preference, nurse's preference, and type of medication to be administered.

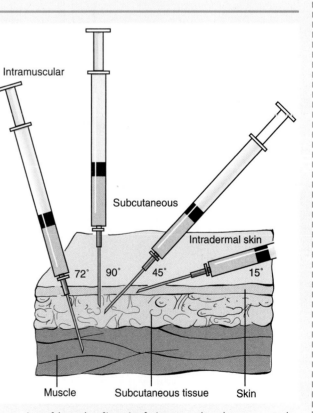

Comparison of the angles of insertion for intramuscular, subcutaneous, and intradermal injections.

continues

BOX 5 **Subcutaneous Injections** (continued)

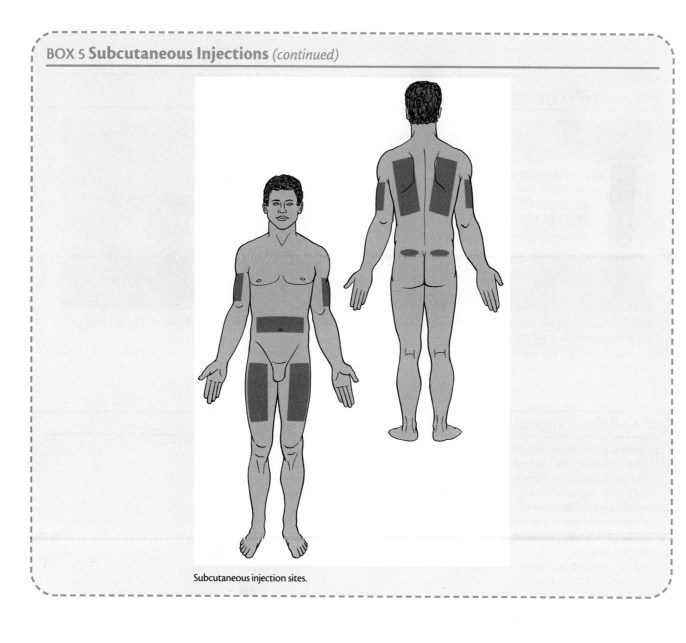

Subcutaneous injection sites.

BOX 6 Intramuscular Site Selection

- Intramuscular injections should contain no more than 3 to 5 mL. The smaller the muscle being injected, the smaller the amount should be.
- The normal angle of insertion for an intramuscular injection is 72 to 90 degrees. This angle depends on the length of the needle and the amount of adipose tissue the patient has (see Box 3).
- Intramuscular injection sites include:
  - Vastus lateralis
  - Ventrogluteal
  - Deltoid
  - Dorsogluteal

- Insertion site selection depends on:
  - Amount of medication
  - Viscosity of medication
  - Age of patient/development of muscle tissue
  - Preference of patient and nurse
  - Ability of patient to assume position needed for injection
- The ventrogluteal site is the most frequently recommended IM injection site for patients over 7 months old because the muscle is well developed and the site is free of nerves and blood vessels and easily identifiable by bony landmarks.

Intramuscular injection sites. (**A**) Ventrogluteal. (**B**) Vastus lateralis. (**C**) Deltoid muscle. (**D**) Dorsogluteal.

Administering Oral Medications

The oral route is the most commonly used route. Drugs given orally are intended for absorption in the stomach and small intestine.

Equipment

- Medication in disposable cup or oral syringe
- Liquid with straw if not contraindicated
- Medication cart or tray
- Medication Kardex or computer-generated MAR

ASSESSMENT

Assess the patient's ability to swallow medications. If the patient cannot swallow, is NPO, or is experiencing nausea or vomiting, the medication should be withheld, the physician notified, and proper documentation completed. Assess the patient's knowledge of the medication. If the patient has a knowledge deficit about the medication, this may be the appropriate time to begin education about the medication. If the medication may affect the patient's vital signs, assess them before administration. If the medication is for pain relief, assess the patient's pain level before and after administration.

NURSING DIAGNOSIS

Determine related factors for the nursing diagnoses based on the patient's current status. Appropriate nursing diagnoses may include:

- Impaired Swallowing
- Risk for Aspiration
- Anxiety
- Deficient Knowledge
- Noncompliance

OUTCOME IDENTIFICATION AND PLANNING

The expected outcome to achieve when administering an oral medication is that the patient will swallow the medication. Other outcomes that may be appropriate include the following: the patient will not aspirate; the patient has decreased anxiety; and the patient understands and complies with the medication regimen.

IMPLEMENTATION

ACTION	RATIONALE
1. Gather equipment. Check each medication order against the original physician's order according to agency policy. Clarify any inconsistencies. Check the patient's chart for allergies.	This comparison helps to identify errors that may have occurred when orders were transcribed. The physician's order is the legal record of medication orders for each agency.
2. Know the actions, special nursing considerations, safe dose ranges, purpose of administration, and adverse effects of the medications to be administered.	This knowledge aids the nurse in evaluating the therapeutic effect of the medication in relation to the patient's disorder and can also be used to educate the patient about the medication.
3. Perform hand hygiene.	Hand hygiene prevents the spread of microorganisms.
4. Move the medication cart to the outside of the patient's room or prepare for administration in the medication area.	Organization facilitates error-free administration and saves time.
5. Unlock the medication cart or drawer.	Locking of the cart or drawer safeguards each patient's medication supply. Hospital accrediting organizations require medication carts to be locked when not in use.
6. **Prepare medications for one patient at a time.**	This prevents errors in medication administration.
7. Select the proper medication from the drawer or stock and compare with the Kardex or order. Check expiration dates and perform calculations if necessary.	Comparison of medication to physician's order reduces errors in medication administration. This is the first safety check. Verify calculations with another nurse if necessary.

continues

Administering Oral Medications (continued)

ACTION

RATIONALE

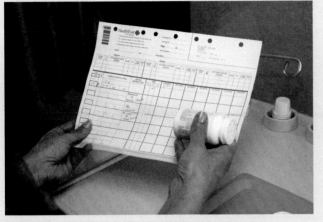

Action 7: Comparing medication with Kardex or order.

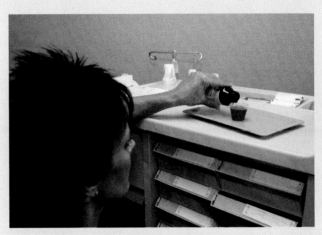

Action 7c: Measuring at eye level.

a. Place unit dose-packaged medications in a disposable cup. **Do not open wrapper until at the bedside.** Keep narcotics and medications that require special nursing assessments in a separate container.

b. When removing tablets or capsules from a bottle, pour the necessary number into the bottle cap and then place the tablets in a medication cup. Break only scored tablets, if necessary, to obtain the proper dosage. Do not touch tablets with hands.

c. Hold liquid medication bottles with the label against the palm. Use the appropriate measuring device when pouring liquids, and read the amount of medication at the bottom of the meniscus at eye level. Wipe the lip of the bottle with a paper towel.

8. **Recheck each medication package or preparation with the order as it is poured.**

9. **When all medications for one patient have been prepared, recheck once again with the medication order before taking them to the patient.**

10. Transport medications to the patient's bedside carefully, and keep the medications in sight at all times.

11. **See that the patient receives the medications at the correct time.**

12. **Identify the patient carefully.** There are three correct ways to do this:

a. Check the name on the patient's identification band.

b. Ask the patient to state his or her name.

a. The label is needed for an additional safety check. Prerequisites to giving certain medications may include assessing vital signs and checking laboratory test results.

b. Pouring medication into the cap allows for easy return of excess medication to bottle. Pouring tablets or capsules into the nurse's hand is unsanitary.

c. Liquid that may drip onto the label makes the label difficult to read. Accuracy is possible when the appropriate measuring device is used and then read accurately.

This is a *second* check to guard against a medication error.

This is a *third* check to ensure accuracy and to prevent errors.

Careful handling and close observation prevent accidental or deliberate disarrangement of medications.

Check agency policy, which may allow for administration within a period of 30 minutes before or 30 minutes after designated time.

Identifying the patient is the nurse's responsibility to guard against error.

a. This is the most reliable method. Replace the identification band if it is missing or inaccurate in any way.

b. This requires a response from the patient, but illness and strange surroundings often cause patients to be confused.

continues

ACTION

RATIONALE

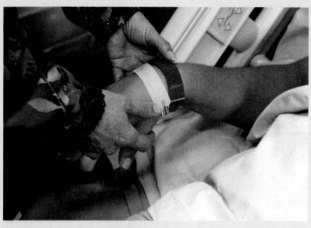

Action 12a: Checking patient identity.

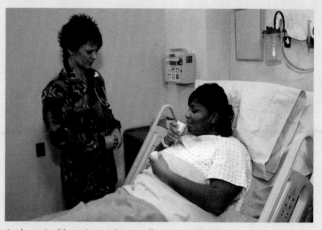

Action 16: Observing patient swallowing medication.

c. Verify the patient's identification with a staff member who knows the patient.

c. This is another way to double-check identity. Do not use the name on the door or over the bed, because these may be inaccurate.

13. **Complete necessary assessments before administering medications. Check allergy bracelet or ask patient about allergies. Explain the purpose and action of each medication to the patient.**

Assessment is a prerequisite to administration of medications.

14. Assist the patient to an upright or lateral position.

15. Administer medications:

Swallowing is facilitated by proper positioning. An upright or side-lying position protects the patient from aspiration.

a. Offer water or other permitted fluids with pills, capsules, tablets, and some liquid medications.

a. Liquids facilitate swallowing of solid drugs. Some liquid drugs are intended to adhere to the pharyngeal area, in which case liquid is not offered with the medication.

b. Ask whether the patient prefers to take the medications by hand or in a cup and one at a time or all at once.

b. This encourages the patient's participation in taking the medications.

c. If the capsule or tablet falls to the floor, it must be discarded and a new one administered.

c. This prevents contamination.

d. Record any fluid intake if intake and output measurement is ordered.

d. This provides for accurate documentation.

16. **Remain with the patient until each medication is swallowed. Never leave medication at the patient's bedside.**

Unless the nurse has seen the patient swallow the drug, the drug cannot be recorded as administered. The patient's chart is a legal record. Only with a physician's order can medications be left at the bedside.

17. Perform hand hygiene.

Hand hygiene prevents the spread of microorganisms.

18. Record each medication given on the medication chart or record using the required format.

Prompt recording avoids the possibility of accidentally repeating the administration of the drug.

a. If the drug was refused or omitted, record this in the appropriate area on the medication record and notify the physician.

a. This verifies the reason medication was omitted and ensures that the physician is aware of the patient's condition.

b. Recording of administration of a narcotic may require additional documentation on a narcotic record, stating drug count and other specific information.

b. Controlled substance laws necessitate careful recording of narcotic use. If a computerized medication station is being used, the machine may document needed information upon withdrawal of the medication.

continues

Administering Oral Medications (continued)

ACTION	RATIONALE

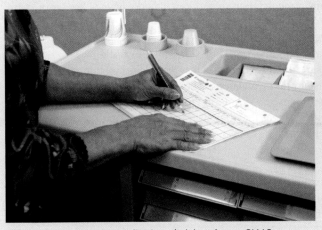

Action 18: Documenting medication administration on CMAR.

> 8/6/06   0835   Mr. Jones complaining of leg pains. Rates pain as an 8/10. 2 Percocet administered.—K. Sanders, RN
>
> 8/6/06   0905   Mr. Jones resting comfortably. Rates leg pain as a 1/10.—K. Sanders, RN
>
> 8/6/06   1300   Mr. Jones refusing to take pain medication. States, "It made me feel woozy last time". Feelings discussed with patient. Patient agrees to take 1 Percocet at this time.—K. Sanders, RN
>
> 8/6/06   1320   Percocet, 1 tablet given P.O. —K. Sanders, RN

Action 19: Documentation.

19. Check on the patient within 30 minutes to verify response to medication.

This provides the opportunity for further documentation and additional assessment of effectiveness of pain relief and adverse effects of medications.

EVALUATION

The expected outcomes are met when the patient swallowed the medication, did not aspirate, has decreased anxiety, and understood and complied with the medication administration.

Unexpected Situations and Associated Interventions

- *Patient feels that medication is lodged in throat:* Offer patient more fluids to drink. If allowed, offer the patient bread or crackers to help move the medication to stomach.
- *It is unclear whether patient swallowed medication:* Check in the patient's mouth, under tongue, and between cheek and gum. Patients may "cheek" medications to avoid taking the medication or to save it for later use. This has been established with many medications, especially antidepressants and pain medication. Patients requiring suicide precautions should be watched closely to ensure that they are not "cheeking" the medication or hiding it in the mouth; they may be trying to accumulate a large amount of medication to take all at once in a suicide attempt. Substance abusers may cheek medication in order to accumulate a large amount to take all at once so that they may feel a high from medication.
- *Patient vomits immediately or shortly after receiving oral medication:* Assess vomit, looking for pills or fragments. Do not readminister medication without notifying physician. If a whole pill is seen and can be identified, physician may ask that medication be administered again. If a pill is not seen or medications cannot be identified, medication should not be readministered so that patient does not receive too large of a dose.
- *Child refuses to take oral medications:* Some medications may be hidden in a small amount of food, such as pudding or ice cream. Do not add to liquid, because medication may alter the taste of liquids; if child then refuses to drink the rest of the liquid, you will not know how much of the medication was ingested. Creativity may be needed when devising ways to administer medications to a child. See below for suggestions.

continues

Administering Oral Medications (continued)

Infant and Child Considerations

- Special devices, such as oral syringes and calibrated nipples, are available in a pharmacy to ensure accurate dose calculations for young children and infants.
- Some creative ways to administer medications to children include: have a "tea party" with medicine cups; place syringe (without needle) or dropper in the space between the cheek and gum and slowly administer the medication; save a special treat for after the medication administration (eg, movie, playroom time, or a special food if allowed).
- The FDA has received reports of infants choking on the plastic caps that fit on the end of syringes when used to administer oral medications. They recommend the following: remove and dispose of caps before giving syringes to patients or families, caution family caregivers to dispose of caps on syringes they buy over the counter, and report any problems with syringe caps to the FDA. Companies have begun to manufacture syringes labeled "oral use" without the caps on them.

Older Adult Considerations

- Elderly patients with arthritis may have difficulty opening childproof caps. On request, the pharmacist can substitute a cap that is easier to open. A rubber band twisted around the cap may provide a more secure grip for older patients.

Home Care Considerations

- Encourage the patient to discard outdated prescription medications.
- Discuss safe storage of medications when there are children and pets in the environment.
- Discuss with parents the difference in over-the-counter medications made for infants and medications made for children. Many times parents do not realize that there are different strengths to the actual medications, leading to under- or over-dosing.
- Encourage patients to carry a card listing all medications, dosage, and frequency in case of an emergency.

Special Considerations

- If the patient questions a medication order or states the medication is different from the usual dose, always recheck and clarify with the original order or physician before giving medication.
- If the patient's level of consciousness is altered or his or her swallowing is impaired, check with the physician to clarify the route of administration or alternative forms of medication. This may also be a solution for a pediatric or a confused patient who is refusing to take a medication.
- Patients with poor vision can request large-type labels on medication containers. A magnifying lens also may be helpful.

SKILL
2

Removing Medication From an Ampule

An ampule is a glass flask that contains a single dose of medication for parenteral administration. Because there is no way to prevent airborne contamination of any unused portion of medication after the ampule is opened, if not all the medication is used, the remainder must be discarded. Medication is removed from an ampule after its thin neck is broken.

Equipment

- Sterile syringe and filter needle
- Ampule of medication
- Needle (optional; for medications that are to be given IM, size depends on medication being administered and patient)
- Antimicrobial swab or gauze pad
- Medication Kardex or computer-generated MAR

ASSESSMENT

Assess the medication in the ampule for any particles or discoloration. Assess the ampule for any cracks or chips. Check expiration date before administering the medication.

NURSING DIAGNOSIS

Determine related factors for the nursing diagnoses based on the patient's current status. Appropriate nursing diagnoses may include:

- Risk for Infection
- Risk for Injury

OUTCOME IDENTIFICATION AND PLANNING

The expected outcome to achieve when removing medication from an ampule is that the medication will be removed in a sterile manner and free from glass shards.

IMPLEMENTATION

ACTION	RATIONALE
1. Gather equipment. Check the medication order against the original physician's order according to agency policy.	This comparison helps to identify errors that may have occurred when orders were transcribed.
2. Perform hand hygiene.	Hand hygiene deters the spread of microorganisms.
3. Tap the stem of the ampule or twist your wrist quickly while holding the ampule vertically.	This facilitates movement of medication in the stem to the body of the ampule.
4. **Wrap a small gauze pad or dry antimicrobial swab around the neck of the ampule.**	This protects the nurse's fingers from the glass as the ampule is broken.
5. Use a snapping motion to break off the top of the ampule along the scored line at its neck. Always break away from your body.	This protects the nurse's face and fingers from any shattered glass fragments.
6. **Remove the cap from the filter needle by pulling it straight off. Insert the filter needle into the ampule, being careful not to touch the rim.**	The rim of the ampule is considered contaminated. Use of a filter needle prevents the accidental withdrawing of small glass particles with the medication.
7. Withdraw medication in the amount ordered plus a small amount more (approximately 30%). **Do not inject air into solutions.** Use either of the following methods:	By withdrawing a small amount more of medication, any air bubbles in the syringe can be displaced once the syringe is removed and there will still be ample medication in the syringe.
a. Insert the tip of the needle into the ampule, which is upright on a flat surface, and withdraw fluid into the syringe. **Touch plunger at knob only.**	a. The contents of the ampule are not under pressure; therefore, air is unnecessary and will cause the contents to overflow. Handling plunger at knob only will keep shaft of plunger sterile.

continues

Removing Medication From an Ampule (continued)

ACTION	RATIONALE

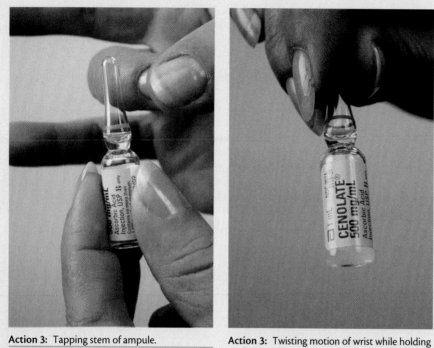

Action 3: Tapping stem of ampule.

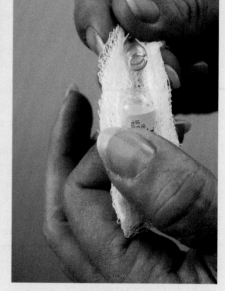

Action 3: Twisting motion of wrist while holding ampule.

Action 4: Snapping off top of ampule.

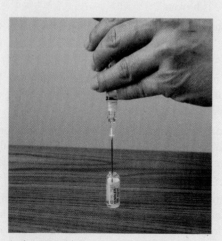

Action 7a: Withdrawing medication from upright ampule.

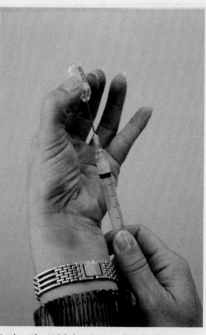

Action 7b: Withdrawing medication from inverted ampule.

continues

Removing Medication From an Ampule (continued)

ACTION

RATIONALE

b. Insert the tip of the needle into the ampule and invert the ampule. Keep the needle centered and not touching the sides of the ampule. Withdraw fluid into syringe. **Touch plunger at knob only.**

b. Surface tension holds the fluids in the ampule when inverted. If the needle touches the sides or is removed and then reinserted into the ampule, surface tension is broken, and fluid runs out. Handling plunger at knob only will keep shaft of plunger sterile.

8. **Wait until the needle has been withdrawn to tap the syringe and expel the air carefully. Do not expel any air bubbles that may form in the solution. Check the amount of medication in the syringe and discard any surplus.**

Ejecting air into the solution increases pressure in the ampule and can force the medication to spill out over the ampule. Ampules may have overfill. Careful measurement ensures that correct dose is withdrawn.

9. Discard the ampule in a suitable container after comparing with the medication Kardex.

Any medication that has not been removed from the ampule must be discarded because there is no way to maintain sterility of contents in an unopened ampule.

10. **Discard the filter needle in a suitable container. If medication is to be given IM or if agency requires the use of a needle to administer medication, attach selected needle to syringe.**

Filter needle used to draw up medication should not be used to administer the medication, to prevent any glass shards from entering the patient. If agency has a needleless IV system, medication is ready to be given.

11. Perform hand hygiene.

Hand hygiene deters the spread of microorganisms.

EVALUATION

The expected outcome is met when the medication is removed from the ampule in a sterile manner and free from glass shards.

Unexpected Situations and Associated Interventions

- *Nurse cuts self while trying to open ampule:* Discard ampule in case contamination has occurred. Bandage wound and retrieve new ampule. Report according to agency policy.
- *All of medication was not removed from the stem and there is not enough medication left in body of ampule for dose:* Retrieve another ampule for the remainder of the dose. Medication should be considered contaminated once neck of ampule has been placed on a nonsterile surface.
- *Nurse injects air into inverted ampule, spraying medication:* Wash hands to remove any medication. If any medication has gotten into eyes, perform an eye irrigation. Retrieve new ampule for medication dose. Report according to agency policy.
- *Medication is drawn up without using a filter needle:* Replace needle with a filter needle. If medication is to be given IM or agency uses a needleless IV system, medication can be injected into a new syringe and then administered to patient.
- *Plunger becomes contaminated before inserted into ampule:* Discard needle and syringe and start over. If plunger is contaminated after medication is drawn into the syringe, it is not necessary to discard and start over. The contaminated plunger will enter the barrel of the syringe when pushing the medication out and will not contaminate the medication.

Removing Medication From a Vial

A vial is a glass bottle with a self-sealing stopper through which medication is removed. For safety in transporting and storing, the single-dose rubber-capped vial is usually covered with a soft metal cap that can be removed easily. The rubber stopper that is then exposed is the means of entrance into the vial.

Equipment

- Sterile syringe and needle (size depends on medication being administered and patient)
- Vial of medication
- Antimicrobial swab
- Second needle (optional)
- Filter needle (optional)
- Medication Kardex or computer-generated MAR

ASSESSMENT

Assess the medication in vial for any discoloration or particles. Check expiration date before administering medication.

NURSING DIAGNOSIS

Determine related factors for the nursing diagnoses based on the patient's current status. An appropriate nursing diagnosis is Risk for Infection.

OUTCOME IDENTIFICATION AND PLANNING

The expected outcome to achieve when removing medication from a vial is withdrawal of the medication into a syringe in a sterile manner.

IMPLEMENTATION

ACTION	RATIONALE
1. Gather equipment. Check medication order against the original physician's order according to agency policy.	This comparison helps to identify errors that may have occurred when orders were transcribed.
2. Perform hand hygiene.	Hand hygiene deters the spread of microorganisms.
3. Remove the metal or plastic cap on the vial that protects the rubber stopper.	The metal or plastic cap prevents contamination of the rubber top.
4. **Swab the rubber top with the antimicrobial swab.**	Antimicrobial swab removes surface bacteria contamination.
5. Remove the cap from the needle by pulling it straight off. (Some agencies recommend use of a filter needle when withdrawing premixed medication from multi-dose vials.) Draw back an amount of air into the syringe that is equal to the specific dose of medication to be withdrawn.	Before fluid is removed, injection of an equal amount of air is required to prevent the formation of a partial vacuum, because a vial is a sealed container. If not enough air is injected, the negative pressure makes it difficult to withdraw the medication. (Use of a filter needle prevents any solid material from being withdrawn through the needle.)
6. Pierce the rubber stopper in the center with the needle tip and inject the measured air into the space above the solution. (Do not inject air into the solution.) The vial may be positioned upright on a flat surface or inverted.	Air bubbled through the solution could result in withdrawal of an inaccurate amount of medication.
7. **Invert the vial and withdraw the needle tip slightly so that it is below the fluid level.**	This prevents air from being aspirated into the syringe.
8. **Draw up the prescribed amount of medication while holding the syringe at eye level and vertically. Be careful to touch the plunger at knob only.**	Holding the syringe at eye level facilitates accurate reading, and the vertical position makes removal of air bubbles from the syringe easy. Handling plunger at knob only will keep shaft of plunger sterile.

continues

SKILL

3

Removing Medication From a Vial (continued)

ACTION   **RATIONALE**

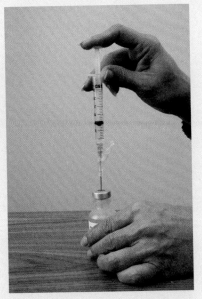

Action 6: Injecting air with vial upright.

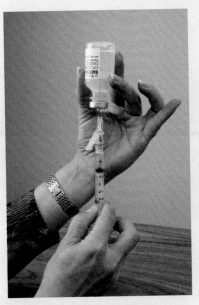

Action 7: Positioning needle tip in solution.

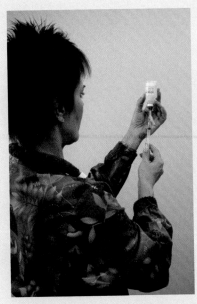

Action 8: Withdrawing medication at eye level.

9. If any air bubbles accumulate in the syringe, tap the barrel of the syringe sharply and move the needle past the fluid into the air space to reinject the air bubble into the vial. Return the needle tip to the solution and continue withdrawal of the medication.

Removal of air bubbles is necessary to ensure accurate dose of medication.

10. After the correct dose is withdrawn, remove the needle from the vial and carefully replace the cap over the needle. If a filter needle has been used to draw up the medication and the medication needs to be administered through a needle, remove the filter needle and replace it with a new needle. (Some agencies recommend changing needles, if needed to administer the medication, before administering the medication.)

This prevents contamination of the needle and protects the nurse against accidental needlesticks. A one-handed recap method may be used as long as care is taken not to contaminate the needle during the process. Filter needle used to draw up medication should not be used to administer the medication to prevent any solid material from entering the patient.

11. **If a multidose vial is being used, label the vial with the date and time opened, and store the vial containing the remaining medication according to agency policy.**

Because the vial is sealed, the medication inside remains sterile and can be used for future injections. Labeling the opened vials with a date and time limits its use after a specific time period.

12. Perform hand hygiene.

Hand hygiene deters the spread of microorganisms.

continues

ACTION   **RATIONALE**

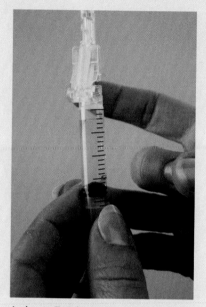

Action 9: Tapping to remove air bubbles.

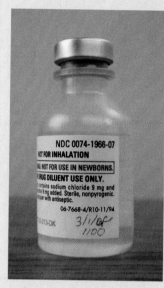

Action 11: Vial with label attached.

EVALUATION

The expected outcome is met when the medication is withdrawn into the syringe in a sterile manner and is ready for administration.

Unexpected Situations and Associated Interventions

- *A piece of rubber stopper is noticed floating in medication in syringe:* Apply a filter needle to the syringe and inject medication into a new syringe. Filter needle should remove any solid material from the medication.
- *As needle attached to syringe filled with air is inserted into vial, the plunger is immediately pulled down:* If possible to withdraw medication, continue steps as explained above. If such a vacuum has formed that this is impossible, remove syringe and inject more air into the vial. This is caused by withdrawal of medication without the addition of air into the vial.
- *Plunger is contaminated before injecting air into vial:* Discard needle and syringe and start over. If plunger is contaminated after medication is drawn into syringe, it is not necessary to discard and start over. The contaminated plunger will enter the barrel of the syringe when pushing the medication out and will not contaminate the medication.

Mixing Insulins in One Syringe

Insulin, a naturally occurring hormone produced by the islets of Langerhans in the pancreas, enables cells to use carbohydrates. Patients with diabetes mellitus type I produce no insulin or produce insulin in insufficient amounts. Several types of insulin are available for use by patients with diabetes mellitus. Insulins vary in their onset and duration of action and are classified as short acting, intermediate acting, and long acting. Many cases of diabetes mellitus are regulated with a combination of two insulins (eg, regular and NPH insulins). Review the duration and peak times of each type of insulin.

Equipment

- Two vials of insulin
- Sterile insulin syringe with 25- to 31-gauge needle
- Antimicrobial swabs
- Medication Kardex or computer-generated MAR

ASSESSMENT

Assess the clarity of each vial of insulin. In the past, clear insulins have been short acting and cloudy insulins have been long acting, but this is no longer the case: there is a new long-acting insulin on the market that is clear. Therefore, it is important to be familiar with each particular insulin's peak and half-life before removing it from the vial.

NURSING DIAGNOSIS

Determine related factors for the nursing diagnoses based on the patient's current status. An appropriate nursing diagnosis is Risk for Infection.

OUTCOME IDENTIFICATION AND PLANNING

The expected outcome to achieve when mixing two different types of insulin in one syringe is that the insulin is appropriately mixed in the syringe in a sterile manner and is ready for administration.

IMPLEMENTATION

ACTION	RATIONALE
1. Gather equipment. Check medication order against the original physician's order according to agency policy.	This comparison helps to identify errors that may have occurred when orders were transcribed.
2. Perform hand hygiene.	Hand hygiene deters the spread of microorganisms.
3. If necessary, remove the cap that protects the rubber stopper on each vial.	The cap protects the rubber top.
4. **If insulin is a suspension (NPH, Lente), roll and agitate the vial to mix it well.**	There is controversy regarding how to mix NPH insulin properly. Some say to roll the vial; others say to shake the vial. Regardless of the method used, it is essential that the suspension be mixed well to avoid administering an inconsistent dose. Regular insulin, which is clear, does not need to be mixed before withdrawal.
5. Cleanse the rubber tops with antimicrobial swabs.	Antimicrobial swab removes surface contamination. It is questionable whether cleaning with alcohol actually disinfects or instead transfers resident bacteria from the hands to another surface. Because it is difficult in a healthcare facility to keep an insulin vial in its original box as recommended, the practice of cleansing with alcohol will most likely continue.
6. Remove cap from needle. Inject air into the modified insulin preparation (eg, NPH insulin). Touch plunger at knob only. Use an amount of air equal to the amount of medication to be withdrawn. **Do not allow needle to touch medication in vial.** Remove needle.	Regular insulin should never be contaminated with NPH or any insulin modified with added protein. Placing air in the NPH insulin first without allowing the needle to contact the insulin ensures that regular insulin is not contaminated with the additional protein in the NPH. Handling plunger by knob only ensures sterility of shaft of plunger.

continues

Mixing Insulins in One Syringe (continued)

ACTION	RATIONALE

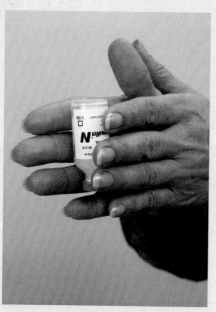

Action 4: Mixing NPH insulin.

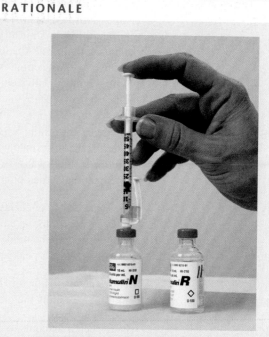

Action 6: Injecting air into modified insulin preparation.

7. Inject air into the regular insulin without additional protein. Use an amount of air equal to the amount of medication to be withdrawn.

An equal amount of air must be injected into the vacuum to allow easy withdrawal of medication.

8. Invert vial of regular insulin and aspirate amount prescribed. Invert and then remove needle from vial.

Regular insulin that contains no additional protein is not contaminated by insulin that contains globulin or protamine.

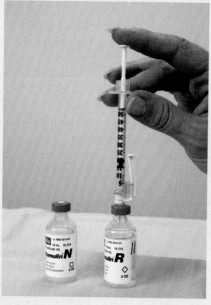

Action 7: Injecting air into regular insulin.

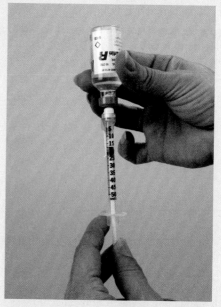

Action 8: Withdrawing regular insulin.

continues

Mixing Insulins in One Syringe (continued)

ACTION	RATIONALE
9. Cleanse the rubber top of the modified insulin vial. Insert the needle into this vial, invert it, and withdraw the medication. Carefully replace the cap over the needle.	Previous addition of air eliminates need to create positive pressure. Capping the needle prevents contamination and protects the nurse against accidental needlesticks. A one-handed recap method may be used as long as care is taken to ensure that the needle remains sterile.
10. Store the vials according to agency recommendations.	Insulin need not be refrigerated but must be protected from temperature extremes.
11. Perform hand hygiene.	Hand hygiene deters the spread of microorganisms.

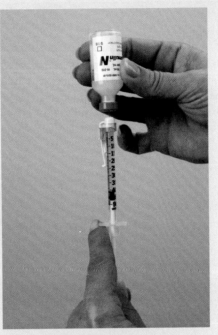

Action 9: Withdrawing modified insulin.

EVALUATION   The expected outcome is met when the insulin is mixed appropriately (in a sterile manner) in the syringe following the steps above and is ready for administration.

Unexpected Situations and Associated Interventions

- *Nurse contaminates plunger before injecting air into insulin vial:* Discard needle and syringe and start over. If plunger is contaminated after medication is drawn into the syringe, it is not necessary to discard and start over. The contaminated plunger will enter the barrel of the syringe when pushing the medication out and will not contaminate the medication.
- *Nurse allows NPH insulin to come in contact with syringe before entering the regular insulin vial:* Discard needle and syringe and start over.
- *Nurse notices that the combined amount is not the ordered amount (eg, nurse has less or more units in combined syringe than ordered):* Discard syringe and start over. There is no way to know for sure which dosage is wrong.
- *Nurse injects regular insulin into NPH vial:* Discard vial and syringe and start over.

continues

Mixing Insulins in One Syringe (continued)

Special Considerations
- An insulin-cartridge pen (the Novolin Pen) is available that allows the patient to dial the correct dose of insulin and press a button to release the dose quickly through a short, fine, 27-gauge needle.
- A type 1 diabetic patient who is visually impaired may find it helpful to use a magnifying apparatus that fits around the syringe.
- Before attempting to explain or demonstrate devices that help low-vision diabetic patients to prepare their medication, attempt to use the device yourself under similar circumstances. To detect any difficulties the patient may experience, practice using the aid with your eyes closed or in a poorly lit room.

Administering an Intradermal Injection

The intradermal route has the longest absorption time of all parenteral routes. For this reason, intradermal injections are used for diagnostic purposes, such as the tuberculin test and tests to determine sensitivity to various substances. The advantage of the intradermal route for these tests is that the body's reaction to substances is easily visible, and degrees of reaction are discernible by comparative study. Intradermal injections are placed just below the epidermis.

Equipment
- Medication
- Sterile syringe and needle (25 to 27 gauge, $\frac{1}{4}''$ to $\frac{5}{8}''$ long)
- Antimicrobial swab
- Disposable gloves
- Acetone and 2×2 sterile gauze square (optional)
- Medication Kardex or computer-generated MAR

ASSESSMENT
Assess the patient for any allergies. Assess the site on the patient where the injection is to be given; it should not be given in broken or open skin. Avoid areas that are highly pigmented and hairy. Assess the patient's knowledge of reason for injection. This may provide an opportune time for patient education.

NURSING DIAGNOSIS
Determine related factors for the nursing diagnoses based on the patient's current status. Appropriate nursing diagnoses may include:
- Deficient Knowledge
- Risk for Allergy Response
- Anxiety

OUTCOME IDENTIFICATION AND PLANNING
The expected outcome to achieve when administering an intradermal injection is appearance of a wheal or blister at the site of injection. Other outcomes that may be appropriate include the following: the patient understands the rationale for the injection; the patient experiences no allergy response; the patient refrains from rubbing the site; and the patient's anxiety is decreased.

IMPLEMENTATION

ACTION	RATIONALE
1. Assemble equipment and check the physician's order.	This ensures that the patient receives the right medication at the right time by the proper route. Many intradermal drugs are potent allergens and may cause a significant reaction if given in an incorrect dose.

continues

SKILL 5

Administering an Intradermal Injection (continued)

ACTION	RATIONALE
2. Explain the procedure to the patient.	Explanation encourages cooperation and reduces apprehension.
3. Perform hand hygiene. Don disposable gloves.	Hand hygiene deters the spread of microorganisms. Gloves act as a barrier and protect the nurse's hands from accidental exposure to blood during the injection procedure.
4. If necessary, withdraw medication from an ampule or vial as described in Skills 2 and 3.	
5. Select an area on the inner aspect of the forearm that is not heavily pigmented or covered with hair. The upper chest and upper back beneath the scapulae also are sites for intradermal injections.	The forearm is a convenient and easy location for introducing an agent intradermally. Hair or lesions at the injection site may interfere with assessments of skin changes at the site.
6. Cleanse the area with an antimicrobial swab while wiping with a firm, circular motion and moving outward from the injection site. Allow the skin to dry. If the skin is oily, clean the area with a pledget moistened with acetone.	Pathogens on the skin can be forced into the tissues by the needle. Introducing alcohol into tissues irritates the tissues and is uncomfortable for the patient. Acetone is effective for removing oily substances from the skin.
7. Remove the needle cap with the nondominant hand by pulling it straight off.	Taut skin provides an easy entrance into intradermal tissue.
8. Use the nondominant hand to spread the skin taut over the injection site.	The cap protects the needle from contact with microorganisms. This technique lessens the risk of an accidental needlestick.
9. **Place the needle almost flat against the patient's skin, bevel side up, and insert the needle into the skin so that the point of the needle can be seen through the skin. Insert the needle only about $\frac{1}{8}$" with entire bevel under the skin.**	Intradermal tissue is entered when the needle is held as nearly parallel to the skin as possible and is inserted about $\frac{1}{8}$".
10. Slowly inject the agent while watching for a small wheal or blister to appear. If none appears, withdraw the needle to ensure bevel is in interdermal tissue.	If a small wheal or blister appears, the agent is in the intradermal tissue.
11. Once the agent has been injected, withdraw the needle quickly at the same angle that it was inserted.	Withdrawing the needle quickly and at the angle at which it entered the skin minimizes tissue damage and discomfort for the patient.

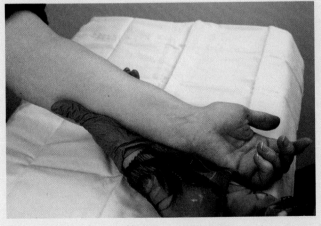

Action 8: Holding forearm skin taut.

continues

Administering an Intradermal Injection (continued)

ACTION

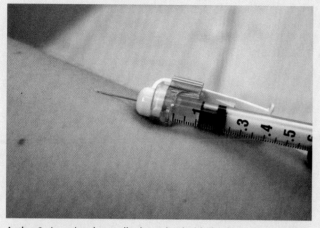

Action 9: Inserting the needle almost level with the skin.

RATIONALE

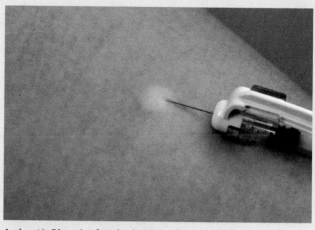

Action 10: Observing for wheal while injecting medication.

12. **Do not massage area after removing needle. Tell patient not to rub or scratch site.**

Massaging the area where an intradermal injection is given may interfere with test results by spreading medication to underlying subcutaneous tissue.

13. Do not recap the used needle. Discard the needle and syringe in the appropriate receptacle.

Proper disposal of the needle protects the nurse from accidental injection. Most accidental puncture wounds occur when recapping needles.

14. Assist the patient to a position of comfort.

This provides for the well-being of the patient.

15. Remove gloves and dispose of them properly. Perform hand hygiene.

Hand hygiene deters the spread of microorganisms.

16. Chart the administration of the medication as well as the site of administration. Some agencies recommend circling the injection site with ink. Charting may be documented on CMAR, including location.

Accurate documentation is necessary to prevent medication error. Circling the injection site easily identifies the site of the intradermal injection and allows for careful observation of the exact area.

17. Observe the area for signs of a reaction at ordered intervals, usually at 24 to 72 hours. Inform the patient of this inspection.

With many intradermal injections, the nurse will need to look for a localized reaction in the area of the injection.

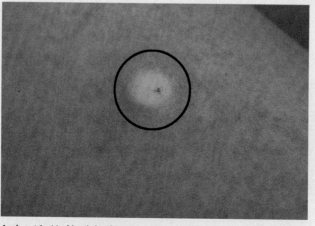

Action 16: Marking injection site.

continues

SKILL
5

Administering an Intradermal Injection (continued)

EVALUATION

The expected outcomes are met when the nurse notes a wheal or blister at site of injection; patient understood the rationale for the injection; the patient experienced no allergy response; the patient does not rub or scratch the site; and the patient's anxiety is decreased.

Unexpected Situations and Associated Interventions

- *Nurse does not note wheal or blister at site of injection:* Medication has been injected subcutaneously. Nurse may need to obtain order to repeat procedure.
- *Medication leaks out of injection site before needle is withdrawn:* Needle was inserted less than ⅛″. Nurse may need to obtain order to repeat procedure.
- *Nurse sticks self with needle before injection:* Discard needle and syringe appropriately. Follow agency policy regarding needlestick injury. Prepare new syringe with medication and administer to patient. Complete appropriate paperwork and follow agency's policy regarding needlesticks.
- *Nurse sticks self with needle after injection:* Follow agency's policy regarding needlestick injuries. Discard needle and syringe appropriately. Complete the appropriate paperwork. Do not document needlestick in patient's notes.
- *After or during injection, the patient pulls away from the needle before medication is delivered fully:* Remove and appropriately discard needle. Attach a new needle to the syringe and administer the remaining medication.

Special Considerations

- Since the needle is entering only the dermal portion of tissue, where there are no large blood vessels, aspiration (pulling back on the plunger) is not recommended for an intradermal injection.
- Some agencies recommend administering intradermal injections with the bevel down instead of the bevel up.

SKILL
6

Administering a Subcutaneous Injection

Subcutaneous tissue lies between the epidermis and the muscle. Because there is subcutaneous tissue all over the body, various sites are used for subcutaneous injections. These sites are the outer aspect of the upper arm, the abdomen (from below the costal margin to the iliac crests), the anterior aspects of the thigh, the upper back, and the upper ventral or dorsogluteal area (see Box 5). This route is used to administer insulin, heparin, and certain immunizations. If needed, review the specifics of the particular medication before administrating.

Equipment

- Medication
- Sterile syringe and needle (size depends on medication being administered and patient)
- Antimicrobial swabs
- Disposable gloves
- Medication Kardex or computer-generated MAR
- Cotton balls or dry sponge (optional)

ASSESSMENT

Assess the patient for any allergies. Assess the patient's knowledge of the medication. If the patient has a knowledge deficit about the medication, this may be an appropriate time to begin education about the medication. Assess the area where injection is to be given. Subcutaneous injections should not be given into areas of skin that are broken or open.

NURSING DIAGNOSIS

Determine related factors for the nursing diagnoses based on the patient's current status. Appropriate nursing diagnoses may include:

- Deficient Knowledge
- Acute Pain
- Anxiety
- Risk for Allergy Response

continues

OUTCOME IDENTIFICATION AND PLANNING

The expected outcome to achieve when administering a subcutaneous injection is that the patient receives medication via the subcutaneous route. Other outcomes that may be appropriate include the following: the patient understands the reason for the procedure and has minimal pain, decreased anxiety, and no allergic response.

IMPLEMENTATION

ACTION	RATIONALE
1. Assemble equipment and check the physician's order.	This ensures that the patient receives the right medication at the right time by the proper route.
2. Explain the procedure to the patient.	Explanation encourages patient cooperation and reduces apprehension.
3. Perform hand hygiene.	Hand hygiene deters the spread of microorganisms.
4. If necessary, withdraw medication from an ampule or vial as described in Procedures 2 and 3.	
5. Identify the patient carefully by checking the identification band on the patient's wrist and asking the patient his or her name. Close the curtain to provide privacy. Don disposable gloves.	It is the nurse's responsibility to guard against error. Gloves act as a barrier and protect the nurse's hands from accidental exposure to blood during the injection procedure.
6. Have the patient assume a position appropriate for the most commonly used sites. See Box 5. a. Outer aspect of upper arm: the patient's arm should be relaxed and at the side of the body. b. Anterior thighs: the patient may sit or lie with the leg relaxed. c. Abdomen: the patient may lie in a semirecumbent position.	Injection into a tense extremity causes discomfort.
7. Locate the site of choice according to directions given in Box 5. Ensure that the area is not tender and is free of lumps or nodules.	Good visualization is necessary to establish the correct location of the site and avoid damage to tissues. Nodules or lumps may indicate a previous injection site where absorption was inadequate.
8. Clean the area around the injection site with an antimicrobial swab. Use a firm, circular motion while moving outward from the injection site. Allow area to dry.	Friction helps to clean the skin. A clean area is contaminated when a soiled object is rubbed over its surface.
9. Remove the needle cap with the nondominant hand, pulling it straight off.	The cap protects the needle from contact with microorganisms. This technique lessens the risk of an accidental needlestick.
10. Grasp and bunch the area surrounding the injection site or spread the skin at the site.	This provides for easy, less painful entry into the subcutaneous tissue. The decision to pinch or spread tissue at the injection site depends on the size of the patient. If the patient is thin, skin needs to be bunched to create a skin fold.

continues

ACTION

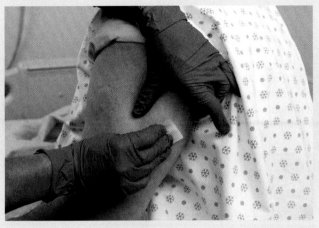

Action 8: Cleaning injection site.

11. **Hold the syringe in the dominant hand between the thumb and forefinger. Inject the needle quickly at an angle at 45 to 90 degrees, depending on the amount and turgor of the tissue and the length of the needle, as shown.**

12. After the needle is in place, release the tissue. If you have a large skin fold pinched up, ensure that the needle stays in place as the skin is released. Immediately move your nondominant hand to steady the lower end of the syringe. Slide your dominant hand to the tip of the barrel.

13. **Aspirate, if recommended, by pulling back gently on the plunger of the syringe to determine whether the needle is in a blood vessel. If blood appears, the needle should be withdrawn, the medication syringe and needle discarded, and a new syringe with new medication prepared.** *Do not aspirate when giving insulin or any form of heparin.*

RATIONALE

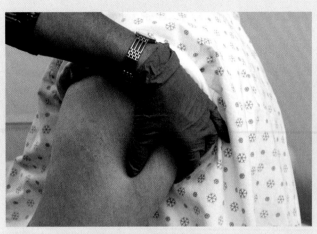

Action 10: Bunching tissue around injection site.

Inserting the needle quickly causes less pain to the patient. Subcutaneous tissue is abundant in well-nourished, well-hydrated people and spare in emaciated, dehydrated, or very thin persons. For a thin person, it is best to insert the needle at a 45-degree angle.

Injecting the solution into compressed tissues results in pressure against nerve fibers and creates discomfort. If there is a large skin fold, the skin may retract away from the needle. The nondominant hand secures the syringe and allows for smooth aspiration.

Discomfort and possibly a serious reaction may occur if a drug intended for subcutaneous use is injected into a vein. Heparin is an anticoagulant and may cause bruising if aspirated. Because the insulin needle is so small, aspiration after insulin has proved unreliable in predicting needle placement.

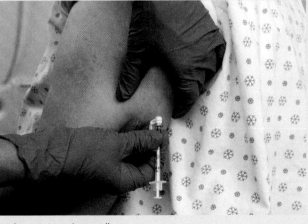

Action 11: Inserting needle.

continues

ACTION	RATIONALE
14. If no blood appears, inject the solution slowly.	Rapid injection of the solution creates pressure in the tissues, resulting in discomfort.
15. Withdraw the needle quickly at the same angle at which it was inserted.	Slow withdrawal of the needle pulls the tissues and causes discomfort. Applying countertraction around the injection site helps to prevent pulling on the tissue as the needle is withdrawn. Removing the needle at the same angle at which it was inserted minimizes tissue damage and discomfort for the patient.

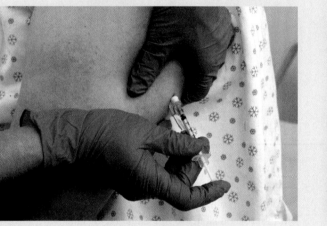

Action 14: Injecting medication.

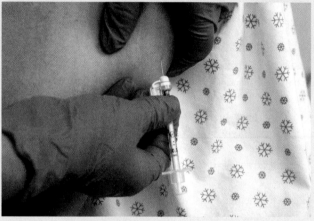

Action 15: Withdrawing needle.

16. Massage the area gently with cotton ball or dry swab. **Do not massage a subcutaneous heparin or insulin injection site.** Apply a small bandage if needed.	Massaging helps to distribute the solution and hastens its absorption. Massaging the site of a heparin injection causes additional bruising. Massaging after an insulin injection may contribute to unpredictable absorption of the medication.

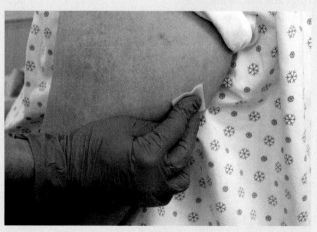

Action 16: Massaging injection site.

continues

Administering a Subcutaneous Injection (continued)

ACTION	RATIONALE
17. Do not recap the used needle. Discard the needle and syringe in the appropriate receptacle.	Proper disposal of the needle protects the nurse from accidental injection. Most accidental puncture wounds occur when recapping needles.
18. Assist the patient to a position of comfort.	This provides for the well-being of the patient.
19. Remove gloves and dispose of them properly. Perform hand hygiene.	Hand hygiene deters the spread of microorganisms.
20. Chart the administration of the medication, including the site of administration. This charting can be done on CMAR.	Accurate documentation is necessary to prevent medication error.
21. Evaluate the response of the patient to the medication within an appropriate time frame.	Reaction to medication given by the parenteral route may occur within 15 to 30 minutes after injection.

EVALUATION

The expected outcomes are met when the patient has received the medication via the subcutaneous route; understands the reason for the procedure; experienced minimal pain; has decreased anxiety; and has had no allergic response.

Unexpected Situations and Associated Interventions

- *When skin fold is released, needle pulls out of skin:* Remove and appropriately discard needle. Attach new needle to syringe and administer injection.
- *Patient refuses to let nurse administer medication in another location:* Explain the rationale behind rotating injection sites. Discuss other available injection sites with patient. If patient will still not allow injection in another area, administer medication to patient, document patient's refusal and discussion, and notify physician.
- *Nurse sticks self with needle before injection:* Discard needle and syringe appropriately. Follow the agency's policy regarding needlesticks. Prepare a new syringe with medication and administer to patient. Complete appropriate paperwork.
- *Nurse sticks self with needle after injection:* Discard needle and syringe appropriately. Follow agency's policy regarding needlesticks. Complete appropriate paperwork. Do not document needlestick in patient's notes.
- *After or during injection, patient pulls away from needle before medication is delivered fully:* Remove and appropriately discard needle. Attach a new needle to syringe and administer remaining medication.

Infant and Child Considerations

- Do not tell a child that an injection will not hurt. Describe the feel of the injection as a pinch or a sting. A child who believes you have been dishonest with him or her is less likely to cooperate with future procedures.

Older Adult Considerations

- Many elderly patients have less adipose tissue. Adjust the angle of the needle accordingly. You do not want to inadvertently give a subcutaneous medication intramuscularly.

Home Care Considerations

- According to the American Diabetes Association, reuse of insulin syringes in the home setting appears safe. Once the needle is dull, it should be discarded (usually after 2 to 10 uses).

Administering an Intramuscular Injection

The intramuscular route is often used for drugs that are irritating because there are few nerve endings in deep muscle tissue. If a sore or inflamed muscle is entered, however, the muscle may act as a trigger area, and severe referred pain often results. It is best to palpate a muscle before injection. Select a site that does not feel tender to the patient and where the tissue does not contract and become firm and tense. Avoid nodules, lumps, and scars.

Absorption occurs as in subcutaneous administration but more rapidly because of the greater vascularity of muscle tissue. The amount of 5 mL is considered the maximum to be given in one site for an adult with well-developed muscles, although the patient's size and the site used (eg, deltoid muscle) may necessitate smaller injection (Nicoll & Hesby, 2002).

An important point in the administration of an intramuscular injection is the selection of a safe site away from large nerves, bones, and blood vessels (see Box 6). When care is not taken, common complications include abscesses, necrosis and skin slough, nerve injuries, lingering pain, and periostitis (inflammation of the membrane covering a bone).

The sites for injecting intramuscular medications should be rotated when therapy requires repeated injections. The sites described in this skill may all be used on a rotating basis. Whatever pattern of rotating sites is used, a description of it should appear in the patient's plan of nursing care.

Equipment

- Disposable gloves
- Medication
- Sterile syringe and needle (size depends on medication being administered and patient)
- Antimicrobial swab
- Dry sponge
- Medication Kardex or computer-generated MAR

ASSESSMENT

Assess the patient for any allergies. Assess the patient's knowledge of the medication. If the patient has a knowledge deficit about the medication, this may be an appropriate time to begin education about the medication. Assess the area where the injection is to be given. Intramuscular injections should not be given into areas of skin that are broken or open. If the medication is for pain, assess the patient's level of pain. If the medication may affect the patient's vital signs or laboratory test results, check them before administering the medication.

NURSING DIAGNOSIS

Determine related factors for the nursing diagnoses based on the patient's current status. Appropriate diagnoses may include:

- Deficient Knowledge
- Acute Pain
- Risk for Allergy Response
- Anxiety
- Risk for Injury
- Risk for Impaired Skin Integrity

OUTCOME IDENTIFICATION AND PLANNING

The expected outcome to achieve when administering an intramuscular injection is that the patient receives the medication via the intramuscular route. Other outcomes that may be appropriate include the following: the patient understands the reasons for the injection; has minimal pain; has no allergy response; has decreased anxiety; and experiences no injury; and patient's skin remains intact.

continues

Administering an Intramuscular Injection (continued)

IMPLEMENTATION

ACTION	RATIONALE
1. Assemble equipment and check the physician's order.	This ensures that the patient receives the right medication at the right time by the proper route.
2. Explain procedure to patient.	Explanation encourages cooperation and alleviates apprehension.
3. Perform hand hygiene.	Hand hygiene deters the spread of microorganisms.
4. If necessary, withdraw medication from an ampule or vial as described in Procedures 2 and 3.	
5. Do not add air to the syringe.	The addition of air to the syringe is potentially dangerous and may result in an overdose of medication.

6. Identify the patient carefully. There are three correct ways to do this:
  a. Check the name on the patient's identification badge.
 	
  b. Ask the patient his or her name.
 	
  c. Verify the patient's identification with a staff member who knows the patient.
	Identifying the patient is the nurse's responsibility to guard against error.
	  a. This is the most reliable method. Replace the identification band if it is missing or inaccurate in any way.
	  b. This requires a response from the patient, but illness and strange surroundings often cause patients to be confused.
	  c. This is another way to double-check identity. Do not use the name on the door or over the bed, because these may be inaccurate.

7. Provide for privacy. Have the patient assume a position appropriate for the site selected, and encourage the patient to relax.
  a. Ventrogluteal: the patient may lie on the back or side with the hip and knee flexed.
  b. Vastus lateralis: the patient may lie on the back or may assume a sitting position.
  c. Deltoid: the patient may sit or lie with arm relaxed.
  d. Dorsogluteal: the patient may lie prone with toes pointing inward or on the side with the upper leg flexed and placed in front of the lower leg.
	Injection into a tense muscle causes discomfort.

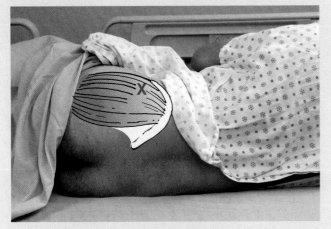

Action 7a: Positioning for ventrogluteal site injection.

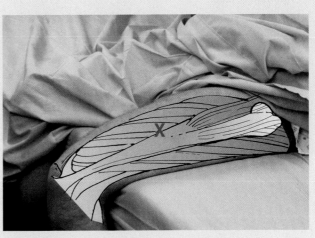

Action 7b: Positioning for vastus lateralis site injection.

continues

Administering an Intramuscular Injection (continued)

ACTION

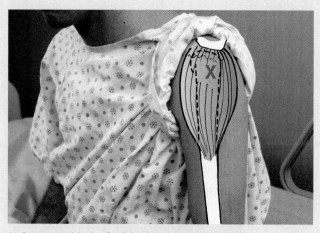

Action 7c: Positioning for deltoid muscle site injection.

RATIONALE

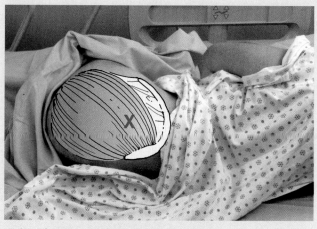

Action 7d: Positioning for dorsogluteal site injection.

8. Locate the site of choice according to directions given in Box 6. Ensure that the area is nontender and free of lumps or nodules. Don disposable gloves.

Good visualization is necessary to establish the correct location of the site and avoid damage to tissues. Nodules or lumps may indicate a previous injection site where absorption was inadequate. Gloves act as a barrier and protect the nurse's hands from accidental exposure to blood during the injection procedure.

9. Clean the area thoroughly with an antimicrobial swab, using friction. Allow to dry.

Pathogens present on the skin and antimicrobial agent can be forced into the tissues by the needle.

10. Remove the needle cap by pulling it straight off.

The cap protects the needle from contact with microorganisms. This technique lessens the risk of an accidental needlestick and also prevents inadvertently unscrewing the needle from the barrel of the syringe.

11. Displace the skin in a Z-track manner by pulling to one side or spread the skin at the site using your non-dominant hand.

This makes the tissue taut and minimizes discomfort. Using the Z-track method prevents seepage of the medication into the needle track and is less painful.

12. Hold the syringe in your dominant hand between the thumb and forefinger. Quickly dart the needle into the tissue at a 90-degree angle.

A quick injection is less painful. Inserting the needle at a 90-degree angle facilitates entry into muscle tissue.

13. As soon as the needle is in place, use your nondominant hand to hold the lower end of the syringe. Slide your dominant hand to the tip of the barrel.

This acts to steady the syringe and allows for smooth aspiration.

14. **Aspirate by slowly (for at least 5 seconds) pulling back on the plunger to determine whether the needle is in a blood vessel. If blood is aspirated, discard the needle, syringe, and medication, prepare a new sterile setup, and inject another site.**

Discomfort and possibly a serious reaction may occur if a drug intended for intramuscular use is injected into a vein. Allowing slow aspiration facilitates backflow of blood even if needle is in a small, low-flow blood vessel.

continues

Administering an Intramuscular Injection (continued)

ACTION   **RATIONALE**

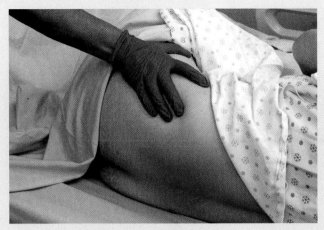

Action 11: Spreading the skin at ventrogluteal site.

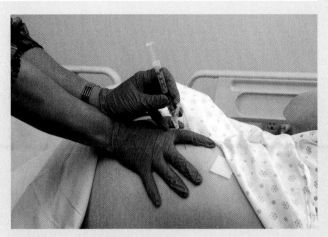

Action 12: Darting needle into the tissue.

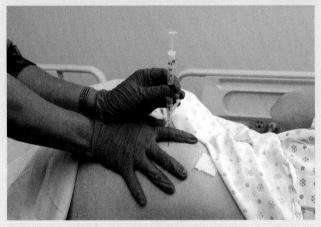

Action 12: Inserting needle in the ventrogluteal site.

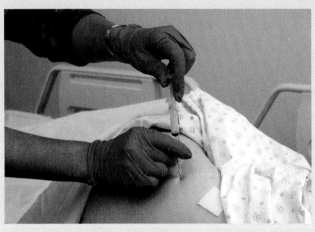

Action 14: Aspirating.

15. If no blood is aspirated, inject the solution slowly (10 seconds per mL of medication).

Injecting slowly helps to reduce discomfort by allowing time for solution to disperse in the tissues.

16. Remove needle slowly and steadily. Release displaced tissue if Z-track technique was used.

Slow withdrawal allows the medication to begin to diffuse through the muscle. Releasing displaced skin seals medication in the tissues.

17. Apply gentle pressure at the site with a small, dry sponge.

Light pressure causes less trauma and irritation to the tissues. Massaging can force medication into subcutaneous tissues.

18. Do not recap used needle. Discard needle and syringe in appropriate receptacle.

Proper disposal of needle protects nurse from accidental injection. Most accidental puncture wounds occur when recapping needles.

19. Assist patient to position of comfort. Encourage patient to exercise extremity used for injection if possible.

Exercise promotes absorption of medication.

20. Remove gloves and dispose of them properly. Perform hand hygiene.

Hand hygiene deters the spread of microorganisms.

continues

ACTION   **RATIONALE**

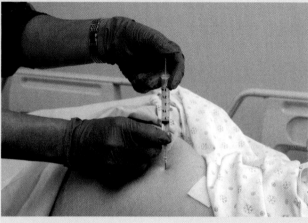

Action 15: Injecting medication.

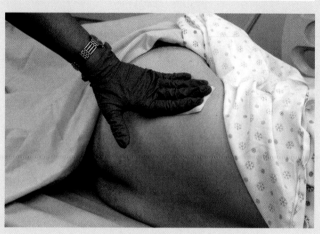

Action 17: Applying pressure at the injection site.

21. Chart the administration of the medication, including the site of administration. This may be documented on the CMAR.

Accurate documentation is necessary to prevent medication error.

22. Evaluate patient's response to medication within an appropriate time frame. Assess site, if possible, within 2 to 4 hours after administration.

Reaction to medication given by the parenteral route is a possibility. Visualization of the site also allows for assessment of any untoward effects.

EVALUATION   The expected outcomes are met when the patient has received the medication via the intramuscular route; understood the reasons for injection; had minimal pain; experienced no allergy response; has decreased anxiety; and experienced no injury; and patient's skin remained intact.

Unexpected Situations and Associated Interventions

- *Nurse sticks self with needle before injection:* Discard needle and syringe appropriately. Follow the agency's policy regarding needlesticks. Prepare a new syringe with medication and administer to the patient. Complete appropriate paperwork.
- *Nurse sticks self with needle after injection:* Discard needle and syringe appropriately. Follow the agency's policy regarding needlesticks. Complete appropriate paperwork. Do not document needlestick in the patient's notes.
- *After or during injection, patient pulls away from needle before medication is delivered fully:* Remove and discard needle appropriately. Attach a new needle to syringe and administer remaining medication in a new site.
- *While injecting needle into patient, nurse hits patient's bone:* Withdraw and discard the needle. Apply new needle to syringe and administer in alternate site. Document incident in patient's notes. Notify physician. May need to complete incident report.

Infant and Child Considerations

- Safe administration of an intramuscular injection into an infant's vastus lateralis muscle may require use of a 1″ needle rather than the commonly used ⅝″ needle. A 1″ needle consistently allows penetration into the muscle and safe administration of the medication.

Adding Medications to an IV Solution Container

Medications may be added to the patient's infusion solution. The recommended procedure is for the pharmacist to add the prescribed drug to a large volume of IV solution, but sometimes the drug is added in the nursing unit, in which case sterile technique must be maintained.

When medication is administered by continuous infusion, the patient receives it slowly and over a long period. Although sometimes this can be an advantage when it is desirable to give the medication slowly, it is a disadvantage when the patient needs to receive the drug more quickly. Also, if for some reason all of the solution cannot be infused, the patient will not receive the prescribed amount of the medication. The patient receiving medication by a continuous IV infusion should be checked for possible adverse effects at least every hour.

Equipment
- Medication prepared in a syringe with a 19- to 21-gauge needle, blunt needle or needleless device (follow agency policy)
- IV fluid container (bag or bottle)
- Antimicrobial swab
- Label to be attached to the IV container
- Medication Kardex or computer-generated MAR

ASSESSMENT
Assess the patient for allergies. Assess the patient's knowledge of the medication. If patient has a knowledge deficit, this may be an appropriate time to begin education about the medication.

NURSING DIAGNOSIS
Determine related factors for the nursing diagnoses based on the patient's current status. Appropriate nursing diagnoses may include:
- Risk for Injury
- Risk for Allergy Response
- Risk for Infection
- Deficient Knowledge
- Anxiety

OUTCOME IDENTIFICATION AND PLANNING
The expected outcome to achieve when adding medications to an IV solution container is that the medication is added to an adequate amount of IV solution and mixed appropriately. Other outcomes that may be appropriate include the following: medication is delivered to the patient in a safe and effective way; patient experiences no allergy response; patient remains infection free; and patient understands and experiences decreased anxiety regarding medication infusion.

IMPLEMENTATION

ACTION	RATIONALE
1. Gather all equipment. Check the medication order with the physician's order and that medication is compatible with IV fluid. Take equipment to patient's bedside.	Checking the order ensures that the patient receives the correct medication at the correct time and in the right manner. Compatibility of medication and solution prevents complications. Having equipment available saves time and facilitates performance of the task.
2. Perform hand hygiene.	Hand hygiene deters the spread of microorganisms.
3. Identify patient by checking identification band on patient's wrist and asking patient his or her name. Check for any allergies patient may have.	This ensures that the medication is given to the right person.
4. Explain procedure to patient.	Explanation allays patient anxiety.

continues

ACTION

RATIONALE

5. Add the medications to the IV solution that is infusing:
   a. **Check that the volume in the bag or bottle is adequate.**
   b. Close the IV clamp.

   c. Clean the medication port with an antimicrobial swab.
   d. Steady the container and uncap the needle or needleless device and insert it into the port. Inject the medication.
   e. Remove the container from the IV pole and gently rotate the solutions.
   f. Rehang the container, open the clamp, and readjust the flow rate.
   g. **Attach the label to the container so that the dose of medication that has been added is apparent.**

   a. The volume should be sufficient to dilute the drug
   b. This prevents backflow directly to the patient of improperly diluted medication.
   c. This deters entry of microorganisms when the port is punctured.
   d. This ensures that the needle or needleless device enters the container and medication can be dispersed into the solution.
   e. This mixes the medication with the solution.

   f. This ensures the infusion of the IV with the medication at the prescribed rate.
   g. This confirms that the prescribed dose of medication has been added to the IV solution.

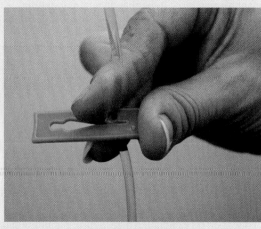

Action 5b: Closing the IV clamp.

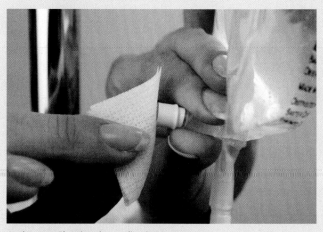

Action 5c: Cleaning the medication port.

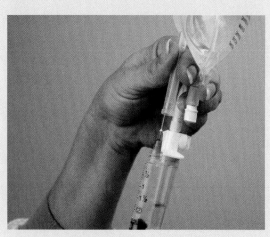

Action 5d: Steadying bag and uncapping needle.

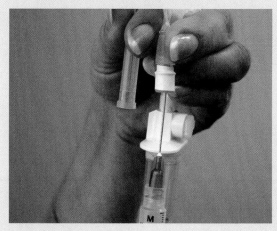

Action 5d: Inserting needle into port.

continues

SKILL 8

Adding Medications to an IV Solution Container (continued)

ACTION

RATIONALE

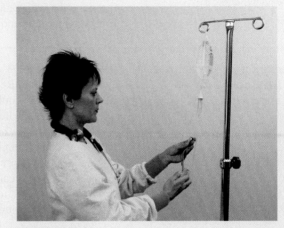

Action 5e: Rotating solution to distribute medication.

Action 5f: Readjusting flow rate.

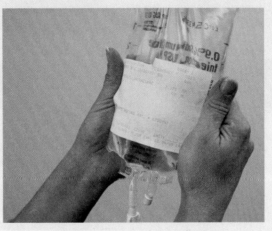

Action 5g: Labeling container to show medication.

6. Add the medication to the IV solution before the infusion:
   a. Carefully remove any protective cover and locate the injection port. Clean with an antimicrobial swab.
   b. Uncap the needle or needleless device and insert into the port. Inject the medication.
   c. Withdraw and insert the spike into the proper entry site on the bag or bottle.
   d. With tubing clamped, gently rotate the IV solution in the bag or bottle. Hang the IV.
   e. **Attach the label to the container so that the dose of medication that has been added is apparent.**

7. Dispose of equipment according to agency policy.

8. Perform hand hygiene.

9. Chart the addition of medication to the IV solution. This may be done on the CMAR.

10. Evaluate the patient's response to medication within the appropriate time frame.

a. This deters entry of microorganisms when the needle punctures the port.
b. This ensures that the needle enters the container and that medication can be dispersed into the solution.
c. This punctures the seal in the IV bag or bottle.

d. This mixes the medication with the solution.

e. This confirms that the prescribed dose of medication has been added to the IV solution.

This prevents inadvertent injury from the equipment.

Hand hygiene deters the spread of microorganisms.

Accurate documentation is necessary to prevent medication errors.

Patients require careful observation because medications given by the IV route may have a rapid effect.

continues

Adding Medications to an IV Solution Container (continued)

EVALUATION

The expected outcomes are met when the medication is added to an adequate amount of IV solution and mixed appropriately; patient received the medication in a safe and effective way; patient experienced no allergy response; patient experienced no infection; patient understood reasons for procedure; and patient experienced decreased anxiety regarding medication infusion.

Unexpected Situations and Associated Interventions

- *There is not enough IV solution in container:* Obtain new IV fluid from medication station and add medication. Remove current IV bag and replace with newly admixed IV fluid. (Some institutions would prefer that the pharmacy mix any new bags so that the process may be done in a sterile environment.)
- *Nurse realizes that wrong medication or wrong amount of medication was added to the IV bag:* Immediately stop infusion. Assess patient for any distress and notify physician. Follow agency policy for medication error. Remove bag of IV fluids and replace with IV containing ordered medication.
- *Nurse sticks self with needle while trying to inject medication into port:* Discard syringe and needle. Prepare new syringe with medication.
- *Needle goes through side of medication injection port:* Discard syringe, needle, and current bag of IV solution. Replace with newly admixed IV fluid. (Some institutions would prefer pharmacy mix any new bags so that the process may be done in a sterile environment.)

Adding a Bolus IV Medication to an Existing IV

A medication can be administered as an IV bolus or push. This involves a single injection of a concentrated solution administered directly into an IV line.

Equipment

- Antimicrobial swab
- Watch with second hand, or stopwatch
- Disposable gloves
- Medication prepared in a syringe with needless device or 23- to 25-gauge, 1″ needle (if needleless system in use, needle is not needed).
- Medication Kardex or computer-generated MAR

ASSESSMENT

Assess patient's IV site, noting any swelling, coolness, leakage of fluid from IV site, or pain. If fluids are infusing through the IV, assess fluid's compatibility with medication to be administered and determine rate at which medication is to be given. Assess patient for allergies. Assess patient's knowledge of medication. If patient has a knowledge deficit, this may be an appropriate time to begin education about the medication.

NURSING DIAGNOSIS

Determine related factors for the nursing diagnoses based on the patient's current status. Appropriate nursing diagnoses may include:

- Acute Pain
- Risk for Allergy Response
- Deficient Knowledge
- Risk for Infection
- Anxiety

Adding a Bolus IV Medication to an Existing IV (continued)

OUTCOME IDENTIFICATION AND PLANNING

The expected outcome to achieve when adding a bolus IV medication to an existing IV is that the IV bolus is given safely. Other outcomes that may be appropriate include the following: patient experiences no or minimal discomfort; patient experiences no allergy response; patient is knowledgeable about medication being added by bolus IV; patient remains infection free; and patient has no, or decreased, anxiety.

IMPLEMENTATION

ACTION	RATIONALE
1. Bring equipment to patient's bedside. Check the medication order with the physician's order. Check a drug resource to clarify whether medication needs to be diluted before administration.	Having equipment available saves time and facilitates performance of the task. Checking the order ensures that the patient receives the correct medication at the correct time and in the right manner.
2. Explain procedure to patient.	Explanation allays patient anxiety.
3. Perform hand hygiene. Don clean gloves.	Hand hygiene deters the spread of microorganisms. Gloves protect the nurse from exposure to bloodborne pathogens.
4. Identify patient by checking the identification band on patient's wrist and asking patient his or her name.	This ensures that medication is given to right person.
5. **Assess IV site for presence of inflammation or infiltration.**	IV medication must be given directly into a vein for safe administration.
6. Select injection port on tubing that is closest to venipuncture site. Clean port with antimicrobial swab.	Using port closest to needle insertion site minimizes dilution of medication. Cleaning deters entry of microorganisms when port is punctured.
7. Uncap syringe. Steady port with your nondominant hand while inserting needleless device or needle into center of port.	This supports injection port and lessens risk for accidentally dislodging IV or entering port incorrectly.

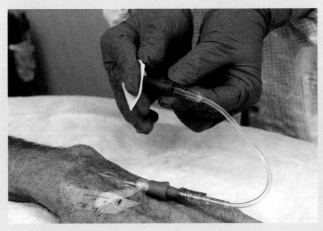

Action 6: Cleaning injection port.

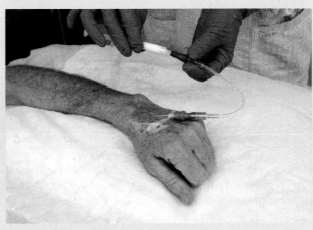

Action 7: Inserting needleless system into port.

8. Move your nondominant hand to section of IV tubing directly behind or just distal to injection port. Fold tubing between your fingers to temporarily stop flow of IV solution.	This minimizes dilution of IV medication with IV solution.
9. Pull back slightly on plunger just until blood appears in tubing. If no blood appears, medication may still be administered while assessing IV insertion site for signs of infiltration.	This ensures injection of medication into a vein.

continues

Adding a Bolus IV Medication to an Existing IV (continued)

ACTION

RATIONALE

10. Inject medication at recommended rate (see Special Considerations below).

This delivers correct amount of medication at proper interval according to manufacturer's directions.

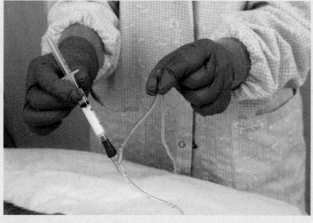

Action 8: Interrupting IV flow.

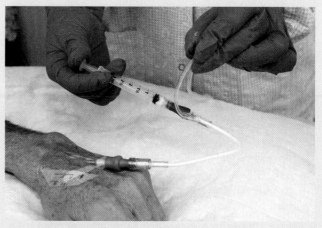

Action 10: Injecting medication while interrupting IV flow.

11. Remove needle. Do not cap it. Release tubing and allow IV to flow at proper rate.

This prevents accidental needlestick.

12. Dispose of syringe in proper receptacle.

Proper disposal prevents accidental injury and spread of microorganisms.

13. Remove gloves and perform hand hygiene.

Hand hygiene deters spread of microorganisms.

14. Chart administration of the medication. This may be done on the CMAR.

Accurate documentation is necessary to prevent medication errors.

15. Evaluate patient's response to medication within appropriate time frame.

Patient requires careful observation because medications given by IV bolus injection may have a rapid effect.

EVALUATION

The expected outcomes are met when the patient receives the medication via an IV bolus; had no, or minimal, discomfort; experienced no allergy response; understood rationale for medication added by bolus IV; experienced no infection; and experienced decreased anxiety.

Unexpected Situations and Associated Interventions

- *Upon assessing patient's IV site before administering medication, nurse notes that IV has infiltrated:* Stop IV fluid and remove IV from extremity. Restart IV in a different location. Continue to monitor new IV site as medication is administered.
- *While administering medication, nurse notes a cloudy, white substance forming in IV tubing:* Stop IV from flowing and stop administering medication. Clamp IV at site nearest to patient. Tubing will need to be flushed thoroughly to get rid of any remaining precipitate. Check literature regarding incompatibilities of medications.
- *While nurse is administering medication, patient begins to complain of pain at IV site:* Stop medication. Assess IV site for any signs of infiltration or phlebitis. You may want to flush the IV with normal saline to check for patency. If the IV site appears within normal limits, resume medication administration at a slower rate.

continues

Adding a Bolus IV Medication to an Existing IV (continued)

Special Considerations

- Agency policy may recommend the following variations when injecting a bolus IV medication:
  - Release folded tubing after each increment of the drug has been administered at prescribed rate to facilitate delivery of medication.
  - Use a syringe with 1 mL normal saline to flush tubing after an IV bolus is delivered to ensure that residual medication in tubing is not delivered too rapidly.
- Consider how fast IV fluid is flowing to determine whether a flush of normal saline is in order after administering medication. If IV fluid is flowing less than 50 mL per hour, it may take medication up to 30 minutes to reach patient. This depends on what type of tubing is being used in the agency.
- If the IV is a small gauge (22 to 24 gauge) placed in a small vein, a blood return may not occur even if IV is intact. Also, patient may complain of stinging and pain at site while medication is being administered due to irritation of vein. Placing a warm pack over vein or slowing the rate may relieve discomfort.

Administering IV Medications by Piggyback, Mini-infusion Pump, or Volume-Control Administration Set

Medications can be administered by intermittent IV infusion. The drug is mixed with a small amount of the IV solution (50 to 100 mL) and administered over a short period at the prescribed interval (eg, every 4 hours). Needleless devices (recommended by the Centers for Disease Control and Prevention and the Occupational Safety and Health Administration) prevent needlesticks and provide access to the primary venous line. Either blunt-ended cannulas or recessed connection ports may be used.

A patient with an IV line in place can receive the solution containing the medication by way of a piggyback setup, a mini-infusion pump, or a volume-control administration set (eg, Pediatrol or Volutrol). The IV piggyback delivery system requires the intermittent or additive solution to be placed higher than the primary solution container. An extension hook provided by the manufacturer provides for easy lowering of the main IV container. The port on the primary IV line has a back-check valve that automatically stops the flow of the primary solution, allowing the secondary or piggyback solution to flow when connected. Because manufacturers' designs vary, check the directions carefully for the systems used in your agency. The nurse is responsible for calculating and manually adjusting the flow rate of the IV intermittent infusion or regulating the infusion with an infusion pump or controller.

The mini-syringe pump for intermittent infusion is battery operated and allows medication mixed in a syringe to be connected to the primary line and delivered by mechanical pressure applied to the syringe plunger.

Medications can also be placed in a controlled-volume administration set for intermittent IV infusion. The medication is diluted with a small amount of solution and administered through the patient's IV line. This type of equipment is also used for infusing solutions into children and older patients when the volume of fluid infused must be monitored carefully.

continues

Equipment

- Medication Kardex or computer-generated MAR

For Piggyback or Mini-infusion Pump:

- Gloves (optional)
- Medication prepared in labeled piggyback set or syringe (5 to 100 mL)
- Secondary infusion tubing (microdrip or macrodrip)
- Needleless device, stopcock, or sterile needle (21- to 23-gauge)
- Antimicrobial swab
- Tape
- Metal or plastic hook
- Mini-infusion pump
- Date label for tubing

For Volume-Control Set:

- Gloves (optional)
- Volume-control set (eg, Volutrol, Buretrol, Burette)
- Medication (in vial or ampule)
- Syringe with needleless device attached or a 20- or 21-gauge needle
- Antimicrobial swab
- Medication label

ASSESSMENT

Assess patient for allergies. Assess patient's knowledge of the medication. If patient has a knowledge deficit, this may be an appropriate time to begin education about the medication. Assess patient's IV site, noting any swelling, coolness, leaking of fluid from IV site, or pain. If fluids are infusing through the IV, assess the fluid's compatibility with the medication to be administered.

NURSING DIAGNOSIS

Determine related factors for the nursing diagnoses based on the patient's current status. Appropriate nursing diagnoses include:

- Acute Pain
- Risk for Allergy Response
- Risk for Infection
- Deficient Knowledge

OUTCOME IDENTIFICATION AND PLANNING

The expected outcome to achieve when administering IV medications by piggyback, volume-control administration set, or mini-infusion pump is that the medication is delivered via the parenteral route. Other outcomes that may be appropriate include the following: patient experiences no or minimal discomfort; patient experiences no allergy response; patient remains infection free; and patient understands the rationale for medication administration.

IMPLEMENTATION

ACTION	RATIONALE
1. Gather equipment and bring to patient's bedside. Check the medication order against the original physician's order according to agency policy.	Having equipment available saves time and facilitates performance of the task. Checking the order ensures that the patient receives the correct medication at the correct time and in the right manner.

continues

Administering IV Medications by Piggyback, Mini-infusion Pump, or Volume-Control Administration Set (continued)

ACTION	RATIONALE
2. Identify patient by checking identification band on patient's wrist and asking patient his or her name.	This ensures that the medication is given to the right person.
3. Explain procedure to patient.	Explanation allays patient anxiety.
4. Perform hand hygiene and don gloves.	Hand hygiene deters the spread of microorganisms. Gloves protect the nurse when connecting setup to an existing IV.
5. **Assess IV site for presence of inflammation or infiltration.**	Medication must be administered directly into a vein that is not inflamed to avoid injuring surrounding tissue.

Using Piggyback Infusion

ACTION	RATIONALE
6. Attach infusion tubing to piggyback set containing diluted medication. Place label on tubing with appropriate date and attach needle or needleless device to end of tubing according to manufacturer's directions. Open clamp and prime tubing. Close clamp.	This removes air from tubing and preserves sterility of setup. Tubing for piggyback setup may be used for 48 to 72 hours, depending on agency policy.
7. **Hang piggyback container on IV pole, positioning it higher than primary IV according to manufacturer's recommendations.** Use metal or plastic hook to lower primary IV.	Position of container influences flow of IV fluid into primary setup.
8. Use antimicrobial swab to clean appropriate port.	This deters entry of microorganisms when piggyback setup is connected to port.
9. Connect piggyback setup to: a. Needleless port b. Stopcock: turn stopcock to "open" position	a&b. Needleless systems and stopcock setup eliminate the need for a needle and are recommended by the Centers for Disease Control and Prevention.
c. Primary IV line: uncap needle and insert into secondary IV port closest to top of primary tubing. Use strip of tape to secure secondary set tubing to primary infusion tubing. Primary line is left unclamped if port has a backflow valve.	c. Tape stabilizes needle in infusion port and prevents it from slipping out. Backflow valve in primary line secondary port stops flow of primary infusion while piggyback solution is infusing. Once completed, backflow valves opens and flow of primary solution resumes.
10. Open clamp on piggyback set and regulate flow at prescribed delivery rate or set for secondary infusion on infusion pump. Monitor medication infusion at periodic intervals.	Delivery over a 30- to 60-minute interval is usually a safe method of administering IV medication. It is important to verify the safe administration rate for each drug to prevent adverse effects.
11. Clamp tubing on piggyback set when solution is infused. Follow agency policy regarding disposal of equipment.	This reduces risk for contaminating primary IV setup.
12. Readjust flow rate of primary IV.	Piggyback medication administration may interrupt normal flow rate of primary IV. Rate readjustment may be necessary.

continues

Administering IV Medications by Piggyback, Mini-infusion Pump, or Volume-Control Administration Set (continued)

ACTION   **RATIONALE**

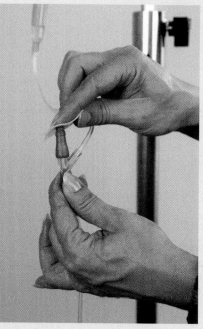

Action 7: Positioning piggyback container on IV pole.

Action 8: Cleaning injection port.

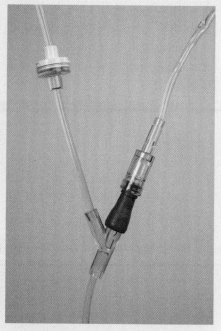

Action 9: Connecting piggyback setup to needleless port.

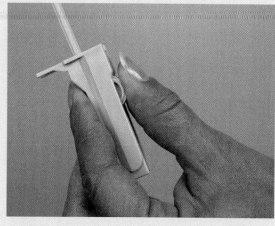

Action 10: Adjusting primary IV fluid to administer piggyback.

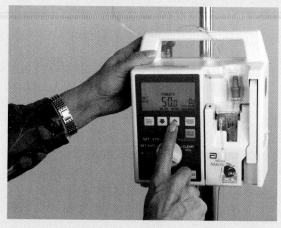

Action 10: Adjusting pump rate.

Using a Mini-infusion Pump

13. Connect prepared syringe to mini-infusion tubing.

14. Fill tubing with medication by applying gentle pressure to syringe plunger.

15. Insert syringe into mini-infusion pump according to manufacturer's directions.

Special tubing connects prepared medication to primary IV line.

This removes air from tubing.

Syringe must fit securely in pump apparatus for proper operation.

continues

ACTION	RATIONALE
16. Use antimicrobial swab to cleanse appropriate connector. Connect mini-infusion tubing to appropriate connector, as in Action 9.	This deters entry of microorganisms when piggyback setup is connected to port. Proper connection allows IV medication to flow into primary line.
17. Program pump to begin infusion. Set alarm if recommended by manufacturer.	Pump delivers medication at controlled rate. Alarm is recommended for use with IV lock apparatus.
18. Recheck flow rate of primary IV once pump has completed delivery of medication.	Normal flow rate of primary IV may have been altered by mini-infusion pump.

Using a Volume-Control Administration Set

19. Withdraw medication from vial or ampule into prepared syringe. See Skill 2 or 3.	The correct dose is prepared for dilution in the IV solution.
20. Open clamp between IV solution and volume-control administration set or secondary setup. Follow manufacturer's instructions and fill with desired amount of IV solution. Close clamp.	This dilutes the medication in the minimal amount of solution. Reclamping prevents the continued addition of fluid to the volume to be mixed with medication.

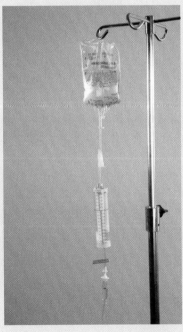

Action 20: Bag with volume control set and tubing.

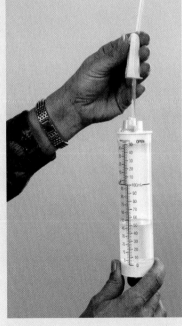

Action 20: Adjusting clamp between bag and volume control set.

21. Use antimicrobial swab to clean injection port on secondary setup.	This deters entry of microorganisms when needle punctures port.
22. Remove clamp and insert needle or blunt needleless device into port while holding syringe steady. Inject medication. Mix gently with IV solution.	This ensures that medication is evenly mixed with solution.

continues

ACTION	RATIONALE
23. Open clamp below secondary setup and regulate at prescribed delivery rate. Monitor medication infusion at periodic intervals.	Delivery over a 30- to 60-minute interval is a safe method of administering IV medication.
24. **Attach the medication label to the volume-control device.**	This prevents medication error.
25. Place syringe with uncapped needle in designated container.	Proper disposal of needle protects the nurse against accidental injection. Most accidental puncture wounds occur when recapping needles.

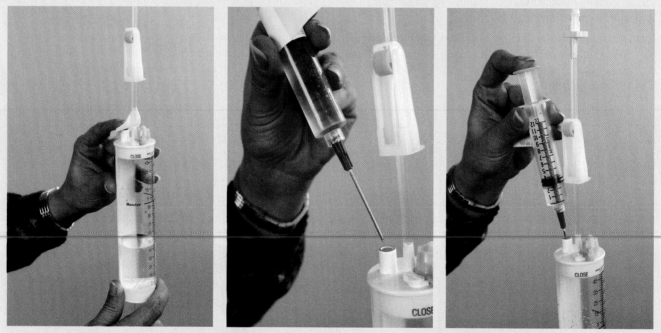

Action 21: Cleaning injection port.

Action 22: Holding syringe steady while inserting blunt needleless device into port and injecting medication.

26. Perform hand hygiene.	Hand hygiene deters the spread of microorganisms.
27. Chart administration of medication after it has been infused. This can be done on the CMAR.	Accurate documentation is necessary to prevent medication errors.
28. Evaluate patient's response to medication within appropriate time frame.	Patient requires careful observation because medications given by the parenteral route may have a rapid effect.

SKILL
10
Administering IV Medications by Piggyback, Mini-infusion Pump, or Volume-Control Administration Set (continued)

ACTION	RATIONALE

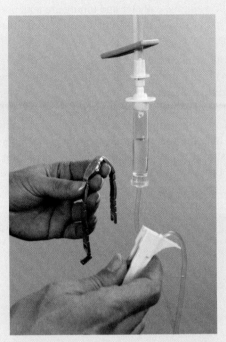

Action 23: Adjusting flow rate of primary fluid.

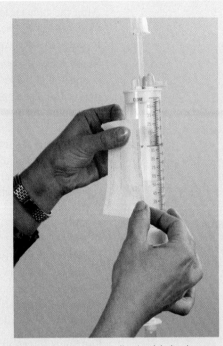

Action 24: Applying medication label to burette.

EVALUATION

The expected outcomes are met when the patient has received the medication via the parenteral route; experienced no, or minimal, discomfort; experienced no allergy response; and experienced no infection; and the patient understood the rationale for medication administration.

Unexpected Situations and Associated Interventions

- *Upon assessing the IV site before administering medication, the nurse notes that the IV has infiltrated:* Stop IV fluid and remove the IV from the extremity. Restart the IV in a different location. Continue to monitor the new IV site as medication is administered.
- *While administering medication, the nurse notes a cloudy, white substance forming in the IV tubing:* Stop the IV from flowing and stop administering the medication to prevent precipitate from entering the patient's circulation. Clamp the IV at the site nearest to the patient. The tubing will need to be flushed thoroughly to rid of any remaining precipitate. Always check the literature regarding incompatibilities of medications before administering.
- *While nurse is administering medication, the patient begins to complain of pain at the IV site:* Stop the medication. Assess the IV site for any signs of infiltration or phlebitis. You may want to flush the IV with normal saline to check for patency. If the IV site appears within normal limits, resume medication administration at a slower rate.

Infant and Child Considerations

- Small infants and children with fluid restrictions may not tolerate the added IV fluid needed for administration with piggyback or volume-control systems. For these children, consider using the mini-infusion pump.

Introducing Drugs Through a Heparin or IV Lock Using the Saline Flush

A heparin or saline lock, or intermittent venous access device, is used for patients who require intermittent IV medication but not a continuous IV infusion. This device consists of a needle or catheter connected to a short length of tubing capped with a sealed injection port. After the catheter is in place in the patient's vein, the catheter and tubing are anchored to the patient's arm so that the catheter remains in place until the patient no longer requires the repeated IV medication.

An IV lock allows the patient more freedom than a continuous IV infusion. The patient is connected to the IV line when it is time to receive the medication and disconnected when the medication is completed. A saline flush rather than a heparin flush is used in many agencies to maintain the patency of the lock. Using saline eliminates any possible systemic effects on coagulation, development of a heparin allergy, and drug incompatibility that may occur when a heparin solution is used. The intermittent infusion is not started until the nurse confirms IV placement. The saline lock is flushed after the infusion is completed to clear the vein of any medication. Positive pressure is used when flushing a saline lock to prevent clot formation in the catheter.

Equipment

- Medication
- Saline vial
- Sterile syringe (two) with needleless device or 25-gauge needle
- Antimicrobial swabs
- Watch with second hand or stopwatch feature
- Gloves (optional)
- Medication Kardex or computer-generated MAR

For Bolus Injection:

- Sterile syringe (two) with needleless device

For Intermittent IV Delivery:

- Needleless device or 25-gauge needle
- IV setup with needleless device attached to tubing or a 25-gauge needle
- Adhesive tape (optional)

ASSESSMENT

Assess the patient for allergies. Assess the patient's knowledge of the medication. If patient has a knowledge deficit, this may be an appropriate time to begin education about the medication. Assess the patient's IV site, noting any swelling, coolness, leaking of fluid from IV site, or pain.

NURSING DIAGNOSIS

Determine related factors for the nursing diagnoses based on the patient's current status. Appropriate nursing diagnoses may include:

- Acute Pain
- Risk for Allergy Response
- Risk for Infection
- Deficient Knowledge

OUTCOME IDENTIFICATION AND PLANNING

The expected outcome to achieve when introducing drugs through a heparin or IV lock using the saline flush is that the medication is delivered via the parenteral route. Other outcomes that may be appropriate include the following: patient experiences no or minimal discomfort; patient experiences no allergy response; patient experiences no infection; and patient understands the rationale for medication administration.

continues

Introducing Drugs Through a Heparin or IV Lock Using the Saline Flush (continued)

IMPLEMENTATION
ACTION

1. Assemble equipment and check physician's order.

2. Identify patient by checking identification band on patient's wrist and asking patient his or her name. Explain procedure to patient.

3. Perform hand hygiene.

4. Withdraw 1 to 2 mL of sterile saline from the vial into the syringe as described in Skill 3.

5. Don clean gloves and prepare to administer medication.

6. **For Bolus IV Injection:**

   a. **Check drug package for correct injection rate for IV push route.**
   b. Clean port of lock with antimicrobial swab.
   c. Stabilize port with your nondominant hand and insert needleless device or needle of syringe of normal saline into port.

RATIONALE

This ensures that the patient receives the right medication at the right time by the proper route.

This ensures that the right patient is receiving the medication. Explanation alleviates the patient's apprehension about IV drug administration.

Hand hygiene deters the spread of microorganisms.

Using saline eliminates concerns about drug incompatibilities and the effect on systemic circulation that exists with heparin.

Gloves protect the nurse's hands from contact with the patient's blood.

a. Using the correct injection rate prevents speed shock from occurring.
b. Cleaning removes surface bacteria at the lock entry site.
c. This allows for careful insertion into the center circle of the lock.

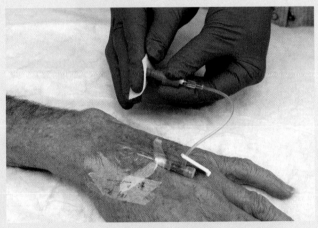

Action 6b: Cleaning port with antimicrobial swab.

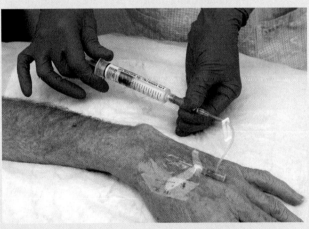

Action 6c: Inserting syringe with blunt needle into port.

d. Aspirate gently and check for blood return (blood return does not always occur even though lock is patent).
e. Gently flush with 1 mL of normal saline. Remove syringe.

f. Insert needleless device or needle of syringe with medication into port and gently inject medication, using a watch to verify correct injection rate. **Do not force the injection if resistance is felt.** If the lock is clogged, it must be changed. Remove medication syringe and needle when administration is complete.

d. Blood return usually indicates that the catheter is in the vein.
e. Saline flush ensures that the IV line is patent. A patient's complaint of pain or resistance to the flush detected by the nurse may indicate that the IV line is not patent.
f. Easy installation of medication usually indicates that the lock is still patent and in the vein. If force is used against resistance, a clot may break away and cause a blockage elsewhere in the body.

continues

ACTION

RATIONALE

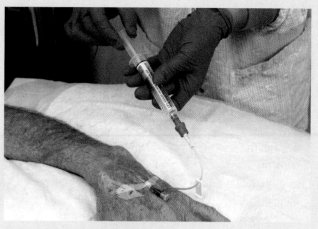

Action 6d: Aspirating for blood return.

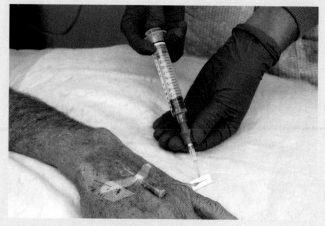

Action 6e: Flushing saline lock.

g. Remove syringe with medication from port. Stabilize port with your nondominant hand and insert needleless device or needle of syringe of normal saline into port. **Slowly flush reservoir with 1 to 2 mL of sterile saline using positive pressure.** To gain positive pressure, you can either clamp the IV tubing as you are still flushing the last of the saline into the IV or remove the syringe as you are still flushing the remainder of the saline into the IV. Remove syringe and discard uncapped needles and syringes in the appropriate receptacle. Remove gloves and discard appropriately.

g. Positive pressure prevents blood from backing into IV catheter and causing the IV to clot off.

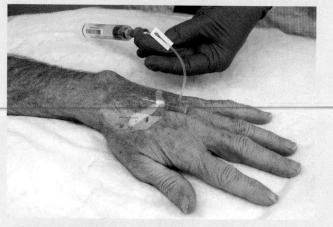

Action 6g: Clamping IV.

7. **For Drug Administration via an Intermittent Delivery System:**

   a. Use a drug resource book to check for the correct flow rate of the medication (the usual is 30 to 60 minutes).

   b. Connect infusion tubing to medication setup according to manufacturer's directions using sterile technique. Hang IV setup on pole. Open clamp and allow solution to clear IV tubing of air. Reclamp tubing.

   c. Attach needleless connector or sterile 25-gauge needle to end of infusion tubing.

   d. Clean port of lock with antimicrobial swab.

   e. Stabilize port with your nondominant hand and insert needleless device or needle of syringe of normal saline into port.

   a. Using the correct injection rate prevents speed shock from occurring.

   b. This removes air from the tubing and preserves the sterility of the setup.

   c. A small-gauge needle prevents damage to the lock.

   d. Cleaning removes surface bacteria at the lock entry site.

   e. This allows for careful insertion into the port.

continues

ACTION

RATIONALE

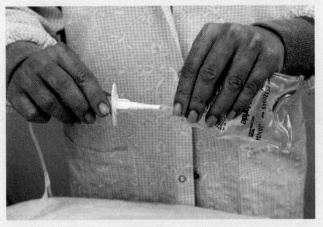

Action 7b: Spiking bag with tubing.

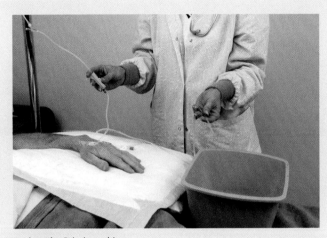

Action 7b: Priming tubing.

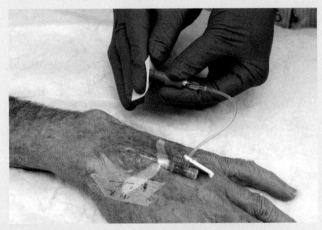

Action 7d: Cleaning port with antimicrobial swab.

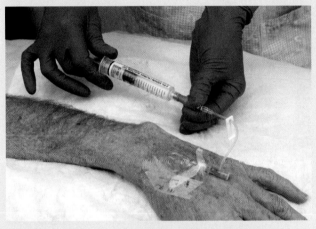

Action 7e: Inserting syringe into port.

f. Aspirate gently and check for blood return (blood return does not always occur even though lock is patent).

g. Gently flush with 1 mL of normal saline. Remove syringe.

h. Insert blunt needleless device or needle attached to tubing into port. If necessary, secure with tape.

i. Open clamp and regulate flow rate or attach to IV pump or controller according to manufacturer's directions. Close clamp when infusion is complete.

j. Remove needleless connector or needle from lock. Carefully replace uncapped, used needle or needleless device with a new sterile one. Allow medication setup to hang on pole for future use according to agency policy. Stabilize port with your nondominant hand and insert needleless device or needle of syringe of normal saline into the port. **Slowly flush the reservoir with 1 to 2 mL of sterile saline using positive pressure.**

f. Blood return usually indicates that the catheter is in the vein.

g. Saline flush ensures that the IV line is patent.

h. Tape secures the needle in the lock port.

i. This ensures that the patient receives the medication at the correct rate.

j. This prevents possible needlestick with contaminated needle. Agency policy specifies length of time for safe use of IV infusion tubing. Saline clears the line of medication with less of the systemic effects of the heparin flush. Positive pressure prevents blood from backing into IV catheter and causing the IV to clot off.

continues

ACTION   **RATIONALE**

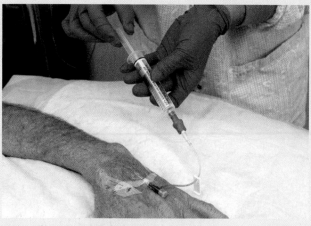

Action 7f: Aspirating for blood return.

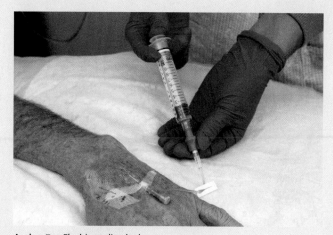

Action 7g: Flushing saline lock.

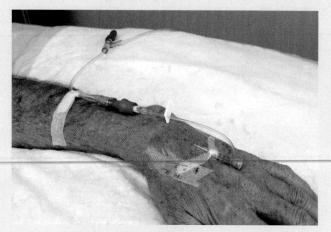

Action 7h: Attaching tubing to saline lock.

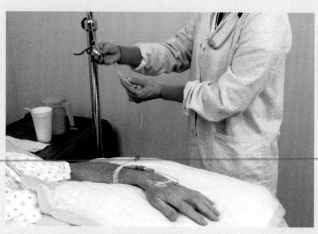

Action 7i: Regulating flow rate manually.

    To gain positive pressure, you can either clamp the IV tubing as you are still flushing the last of the saline into the IV or remove the syringe as you are still flushing the remainder of the saline into the IV. Remove syringe and discard uncapped needles and syringes in appropriate receptacle. Remove gloves and discard appropriately.

8. Perform hand hygiene.

9. Check injection site and IV lock at least every 8 hours and administer a small amount of saline (2 to 3 mL) if medication is not given at least every 8 to 12 hours.

10. **Change heparin lock at least every 72 to 96 hours or according to agency policy.** A lock that is not patent should be changed immediately.

11. Chart administration of medication or saline flush.

Hand hygiene deters the spread of microorganisms.

This ensures patency of system for continuing injections.

Changing a heparin lock regularly and having it free of clotted blood reduces dangers of infection and emboli in the circulating blood.

Accurate documentation is necessary to prevent medication error.

continues

Introducing Drugs Through a Heparin or IV Lock Using the Saline Flush (continued)

ACTION	RATIONALE

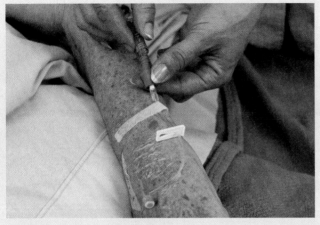

Action 7i: Removing tubing from lock.

EVALUATION	The expected outcomes are met when the patient has received the medication via the parenteral route; experienced no or minimal discomfort; experienced no allergy response; remains infection free; and understood the rationale for medication administration.

Unexpected Situations and Associated Interventions

- *Upon assessing the IV site before administering medication, nurse notes that the IV has infiltrated:* Stop IV fluid and remove IV from extremity. Restart IV in a different location. Continue to monitor new IV site as medication is administered.
- *While nurse is administering medication, patient begins to complain of pain at the IV site:* Stop the medication. Assess the IV site for any signs of infiltration or phlebitis. You may want to flush the IV with normal saline to check for patency. If the IV site appears within normal limits, resume medication administration at a slower rate.
- *Nurse notes white, cloudy particles forming in lock during medication administration:* Stop administering the medication. Remove needle or needleless device from lock. Insert needle or needleless device attached to empty syringe and pull back on plunger, attempting to remove any fluid remaining in lock. If unable to pull back fluid, change lock on IV before resuming medication administration. Entire IV setup and lock may need to be changed.
- *As nurse is attempting to access lock, needle or tip of syringe touches patient's arm:* Discard needle and syringe. Prepare new dose for administration.

Special Considerations

- Some agencies recommend the use of single-dose saline vials without preservative in the solution. Preservatives may be linked to an increased incidence of phlebitis with heparin locks.

Infant and Child Considerations

- If the volume of medication being administered is small (<1.0 mL), always include the amount of flush solution as part of the total amount to be injected and take this into account when determining how fast to push a medication. For example, if the medication is to be injected at a rate of 1.0 mL per minute and the total amount of solution to be injected is 2.25 mL (0.25 mL medication volume plus 2.0 mL saline flush solution volume equals 2.25 ml), then the medication would be injected over a period of 2 minutes 15 seconds.

Instilling Eyedrops

Eyedrops are instilled for their local effects, such as for pupil dilation or constriction when examining the eye, for treating an infection, or to help control intraocular pressure (for patients with glaucoma). The type and amount of solution depend on the purpose of the instillation.

Equipment
- Gloves
- Medication
- Tissue, washcloth
- Medication Kardex or computer-generated MAR

ASSESSMENT

Assess the patient for allergies. Assess the affected eye for any drainage, erythema, or swelling. Assess the patient's knowledge of medication. If patient has a knowledge deficit, this may be an appropriate time to begin education about the medication.

NURSING DIAGNOSIS

Determine related factors for the nursing diagnoses based on the patient's current status. Appropriate nursing diagnoses may include:
- Risk for Allergy Response
- Risk for Injury
- Deficient Knowledge

OUTCOME IDENTIFICATION AND PLANNING

The expected outcome to achieve when administering eyedrops is that the medication is delivered successfully into the eye. Other outcomes that may be appropriate include the following: patient experiences no allergy response; patient's eye remains free from injury; and patient understands the rationale for medication administration.

IMPLEMENTATION

ACTION	RATIONALE
1. Bring equipment to patient's bedside. Check medication order against original physician's order according to agency policy.	Having equipment available saves time and facilitates performance of task. Checking the order ensures that the patient receives the correct medication at the correct time and in the right manner.
2. Identify patient by checking identification band on patient's wrist and asking patient his or her name. Ask patient about any allergies.	This ensures that the medication is given to the right person.
3. Explain procedure to patient.	Explanation allays patient anxiety.
4. Perform hand hygiene and don gloves.	Hand hygiene deters the spread of microorganisms. Gloves protect the nurse when coming in contact with drainage from eyes (solution or tears).
5. Offer tissue to patient.	Solution and tears may spill from the eye during the procedure.
6. **Cleanse the eyelids and eyelashes of any drainage with a washcloth moistened with normal saline solution, proceeding from the inner canthus to the outer canthus. Use each area of the washcloth only once.**	Debris can be carried into the eye when the conjunctival sac is exposed. By using each area of washcloth once and going from the inner canthus to the outer canthus, debris is kept away from the lacrimal duct.
7. Tilt patient's head back slightly. The head may be turned slightly to the affected side.	Tilting patient's head back slightly makes it easier to reach the conjunctival sac. This should be avoided if the patient has a cervical spine injury. Turning the head to the affected side helps to prevent solution or tears from flowing toward the opposite eye.

continues

ACTION

RATIONALE

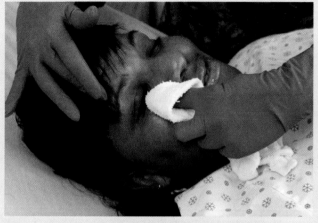

Action 6: Cleaning lids and lashes from inside of eye to outside.

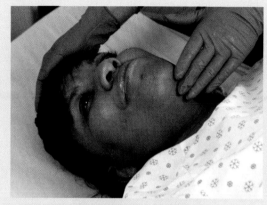

Action 7: Positioning patient for eyedrops.

8. Remove cap from medication bottle, being careful to not touch the inner side of the cap.

9. Invert the monodrip plastic container that is commonly used to instill eyedrops. Have patient look up and focus on something on the ceiling.

10. Place thumb or two fingers near margin of lower eyelid immediately below eyelashes, and exert pressure downward over bony prominence of cheek. Lower conjunctival sac is exposed as lower lid is pulled down.

11. **Hold dropper close to eye, but avoid touching eyelids or lashes. Squeeze container and allow prescribed number of drops to fall in lower conjunctival sac.**

Touching the inner side of the cap may contaminate the bottle of medication.

By having the patient look up and focus on something else, the procedure is less traumatic.

The eyedrop should be placed in the conjunctival sac, not directly on the eyeball.

Touching the eye, eyelids, or lashes can contaminate the medication in the bottle; startle the patient, causing blinking; or injure the eye. Do not allow medication to fall onto cornea. This may injure the cornea or cause the patient to have an unpleasant sensation.

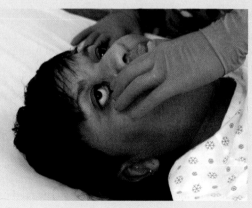

Action 10: Holding eye in position.

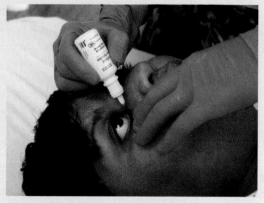

Action 11: Administering eyedrops.

continues

ACTION	RATIONALE
12. Release lower lid after eyedrops are instilled. Ask patient to close eyes gently.	This allows the medication to be distributed over the entire eye.
13. Apply gentle pressure over inner canthus to prevent eyedrops from flowing into tear duct.	This minimizes the risk of systemic effects from the medication.

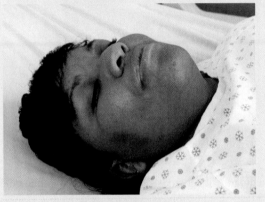

Action 12: Eyes closed.

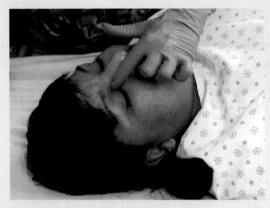

Action 13: Applying pressure.

ACTION	RATIONALE
14. Instruct patient not to rub affected eye.	This prevents injury and irritation to eye.
15. Remove gloves and perform hand hygiene.	Hand hygiene deters the spread of microorganisms.
16. Chart administration of medication. This may be done on the CMAR.	Accurate documentation is necessary to prevent medication errors.
17. Evaluate patient's response to medication within appropriate time frame.	The patient needs to be evaluated for any adverse affects from the medication.

EVALUATION

The expected outcomes are met when the patient has received the eyedrops; experienced no adverse affects, including allergy response or injury; and understood the rationale for the medication administration.

Unexpected Situations and Associated Interventions

- *Drop is placed on eyelid or outer margin of eyelid due to patient blinking or moving:* Do not count this drop in total number of drops administered. Allow the patient to regain composure and proceed with application of medication.
- *Nurse cannot open eyelids due to dried crust and matting of eyelids:* Place a warm wet washcloth over the eye and allow it to remain there for approximately 3 minutes. You may need to repeat this procedure if there is a large amount of matting.
- *Bottle comes in contact with eyeball when applying medication:* Bottle is contaminated; discard appropriately. Notify pharmacy or retrieve new bottle for oncoming shift.

Infant and Child Considerations

- To apply eyedrops in a small child, two or more people may be needed to restrain the child. Make sure the child does not reach up to the eye for fear of jabbing the medication bottle into the eye.

Instilling Eardrops

Drugs are instilled into the auditory canal for their local effect. They are used to soften wax, relieve pain, apply local anesthesia, destroy organisms, or destroy an insect lodged in the canal, which can cause almost intolerable discomfort. If the ear canal has swollen to the point that medication cannot pass, a long piece of cotton material called a wick is inserted so that one end is near the middle ear and the other end is external. This cotton acts as a wick to help medication get to the inner ear.

The tympanic membrane separates the external ear from the middle ear. Normally, it is intact and closes the entrance to the middle ear completely. If it is ruptured or has been opened by surgical intervention, the middle ear and the inner ear have a direct passage to the external ear. When this occurs, instillations should be performed with the greatest of care to prevent forcing materials from the outer ear into the middle ear and the inner ear. Sterile technique is used to prevent infection.

Equipment	• Medication (warmed to 37°C [98.6°F]) • Tissue • Cotton ball (optional) • Gloves (optional) • Washcloth (optional) • Medication Kardex or computer-generated MAR
ASSESSMENT	Assess the affected ear for any drainage or tenderness. Assess the patient for allergies. Assess the patient's knowledge of medication. If the patient has a knowledge deficit about the medication, this may be an appropriate time to begin education.
NURSING DIAGNOSIS	Determine related factors for the nursing diagnoses based on the patient's current status. Appropriate nursing diagnoses may include: • Deficient Knowledge • Anxiety • Acute Pain • Risk for Allergy Response
OUTCOME IDENTIFICATION AND PLANNING	The expected outcome to achieve when administering eardrops is that drops are administered successfully. Other outcomes that may be appropriate include the following: patient understands the rationale for the ear drop instillation and has decreased anxiety; patient remains free from pain; and patient experiences no allergy response.

IMPLEMENTATION

ACTION	RATIONALE
1. Bring equipment to patient's bedside. Check physician's order.	Having equipment available saves time and facilitates performance of task. Checking the order ensures that the patient receives the correct medication at the correct time and in the right manner.
2. Identify patient by checking identification band on patient's wrist and asking patient his or her name. Ask patient regarding any medication allergies.	This ensures that the medication is given to the right person.
3. Explain procedure to patient.	Explanation allays patient anxiety.
4. Perform hand hygiene and don gloves (gloves are to be worn if drainage is present).	Hand hygiene deters the spread of microorganisms. Gloves protect the nurse when coming in contact with drainage from ear.

continues

Instilling Eardrops (continued)

ACTION	RATIONALE
5. Offer tissue to patient.	Solution may spill from the ear during the procedure and run toward the eye.
6. Cleanse external ear of any drainage with cotton ball or washcloth moistened with normal saline.	Debris and drainage may prevent some of the medication from entering the ear canal.
7. Place patient on unaffected side in bed, or if ambulatory, have patient sit with head well tilted to the side so that affected ear is uppermost.	This positioning prevents the drops from escaping from the ear.
8. Draw up amount of solution needed in dropper. Do not return excess medication to stock bottle. A prepackaged monodrip plastic container may also be used.	Risk for contamination is increased when medication is returned to the stock bottle.
9. **Straighten auditory canal by pulling cartilaginous portion of pinna up and back in an adult and down and back in an infant or a child younger than 3 years.**	Pulling on the pinna as described helps to straighten the canal properly for ear drop instillation.

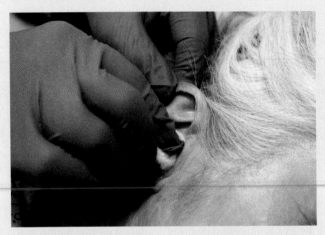

Action 6: Cleaning external ear.

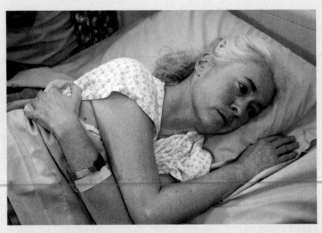

Action 7: Adult positioned for ear drop instillation.

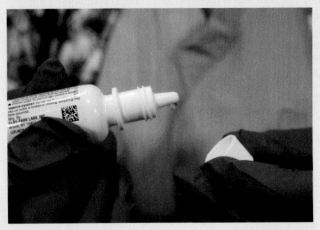

Action 8: Prepackaged ear drop solution.

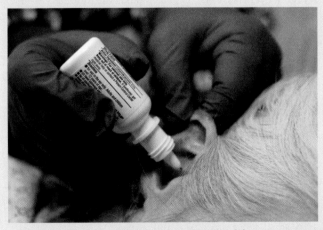

Action 9: Technique for administering ear drops in adult.

continues

SKILL 13 | Instilling Eardrops (continued)

ACTION

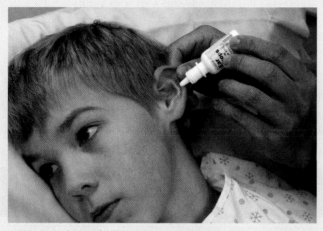

Action 9: Technique for administering ear drops in child over 3 years old.

RATIONALE

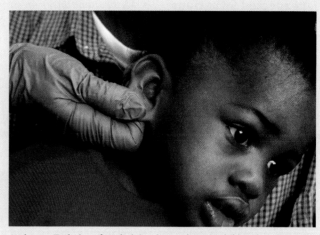

Action 9: Technique for administering eardrops in child under 3 years old.

10. Hold dropper in ear with its tip above auditory canal. For an infant or an irrational or confused patient, protect dropper with a piece of soft tubing to help prevent injury to ear.

11. **Allow drops to fall on side of canal.**

12. Release pinna after instilling drops, and have patient maintain the position to prevent escape of medication.

13. Gently press on tragus a few times.

14. If ordered, loosely insert a cotton ball into ear canal.

15. Remove gloves and perform hand hygiene.

16. Document medication administration and any drainage from ear noted. Documentation may be done on CMAR.

By holding the dropper in the ear, the majority of medication will enter the ear canal. The hard tip of the dropper can damage the tympanic membrane if it is jabbed into the ear.

It is uncomfortable for the patient if drops fall directly onto the tympanic membrane.

Medication should remain in ear canal for at least 5 minutes.

Pressing on tragus causes medication from canal to move toward tympanic membrane.

Cotton ball can help prevent medication from leaking out of ear canal.

Hand hygiene deters the spread of microorganisms.

This provides accurate documentation and helps to prevent medication errors.

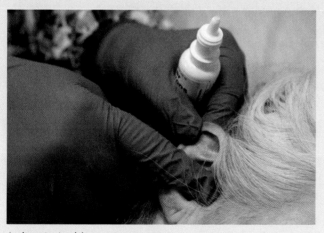

Action 13: Applying pressure to tragus.

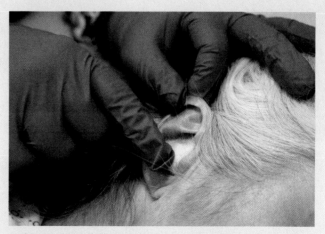

Action 14: Cotton ball inserted in ear.

continues

EVALUATION

The expected outcomes are met when the patient has received the eardrops successfully; understood the rationale for ear drop instillation and exhibited no or decreased anxiety; experienced no or minimal pain; and experienced no allergy response.

Unexpected Situations and Associated Interventions

- *Medication runs from ear into eye:* Notify physician and check with the pharmacy. Eye irrigation may need to be performed.
- *Patient complains of extreme pain when nurse presses on tragus:* Allow patient to press on tragus. If pain is too much, this part may be deferred.

Infant and Child Considerations

- Distraction techniques, such as TV or a quiet toy, may be helpful when attempting to keep a child quiet for 5 minutes. Reading to the child may not be appropriate because the child's hearing may be compromised during medication administration.

SKILL
14
Instilling Nose Drops

Nasal instillations are used to treat allergies, sinus infections, and nasal congestion. Medications with a systemic effect, such as vasopressin, may also be prepared as a nasal instillation. The nose is normally not a sterile cavity, but because of its connection with the sinuses, medical asepsis should be observed carefully when using nasal instillations.

Equipment

- Medication
- Gloves
- Tissue
- Medication Kardex or computer-generated MAR

ASSESSMENT

Assess the patient for allergies. Assess the patient's knowledge of medication. If the patient has a knowledge deficit about the medication, this may be an appropriate time to begin education. Assess the nares for any drainage or broken skin.

NURSING DIAGNOSIS

Determine related factors for the nursing diagnoses based on the patient's current status. Appropriate nursing diagnoses may include:

- Deficient Knowledge
- Risk for Allergy Response
- Risk for Impaired Skin
- Acute Pain

OUTCOME IDENTIFICATION AND PLANNING

The expected outcome to achieve when instilling nose drops is that the medication is administered successfully. Other outcomes that may be appropriate include the following: patient understands the rationale for the nose drop instillation; patient experiences no allergy response; patient's skin remains intact; patient experiences no, or minimal, pain.

IMPLEMENTATION

ACTION	RATIONALE
1. Bring equipment to patient's bedside. Check physician's order.	Having equipment available saves time and facilitates performance of task. Checking the order ensures that the patient receives the correct medication at the correct time and in the right manner.
2. Identify patient by checking identification band on patient's wrist and asking patient his or her name. Also ask patient regarding any medication allergies.	This ensures that the medication is given to the right person.
3. Explain procedure to patient.	Explanation allays patient anxiety.

continues

SKILL 14

Instilling Nose Drops (continued)

ACTION

4. Perform hand hygiene and don gloves (gloves are to be worn if drainage is present).

5. **Provide patient with paper tissues and ask patient to blow his or her nose.**

6. Have patient sit up with head tilted well back. If patient is lying down, tilt head back over a pillow.

7. Draw sufficient solution into dropper for both nares. Do not return excess solution to a stock bottle.

RATIONALE

Hand hygiene deters the spread of microorganisms. Gloves protect the nurse when coming in contact with drainage from nose.

Blowing the nose clears the nasal mucosa prior to medication administration.

These positions allow the solution to flow well back into the nares. Do not tilt head if patient has a cervical spine injury.

Returning solution to a stock bottle increases the risk for contamination of the stock bottle.

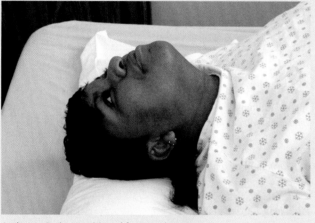

Action 6: Patient positioned for nose drops.

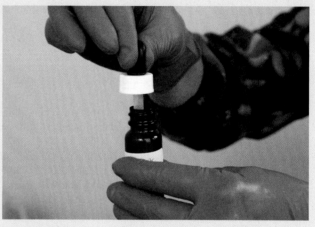

Action 7: Drawing up nose drops.

8. Hold tip of nose up and place dropper just inside naris, about one third of an inch. Instill prescribed number of drops in one naris and then into the other. Protect dropper with a piece of soft tubing if patient is an infant or young child. Avoid touching naris with dropper.

The soft tubing will protect the patient's nares from injury during administration of medication. Touching the naris may cause the patient to sneeze and will contaminate the dropper.

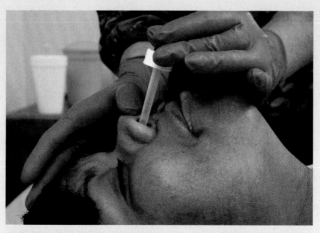

Action 8: Administering nose drops.

continues

Instilling Nose Drops (continued)

9. Have patient remain in position with head tilted back for a few minutes.

Tilting the head back prevents the escape of the medication.

10. Document medication administration and any drainage from nose noted. Documentation may be done on the CMAR.

This provides accurate documentation and helps to prevent medication errors.

EVALUATION

The expected outcomes are met when the patient has received the nose drops successfully; understood the rationale for nose drop instillation; and experienced no allergy response; patient's skin remained intact; and patient experienced no, or minimal, pain or discomfort.

Unexpected Situations and Associated Interventions

- *Patient sneezes immediately after receiving nose drops:* Do not repeat the dosage, because you cannot determine how much medication was actually absorbed.

Bibliography

Abrams, A. (2001). *Clinical drug therapy* (6th ed.). Philadelphia: Lippincott Williams & Wilkins.

Ahmed, D., & Fecik, S. (2000). MAOIs: Still here, still dangerous. *American Journal of Nursing, 100*(2), 29–30.

Carroll, P. (2003). Medication errors: The bigger picture. *RN, 66*(1), 52–58.

Eisenhauer, L., Nichols, L., Spencer, R., & Bergan, F. (1998). *Clinical pharmacology and nursing management* (5th ed.). Philadelphia: Lippincott Williams & Wilkins.

Fain, J. (2002). Delivering insulin round the clock. *Nursing, 32*(8), 54–56.

Fleming, D. (1999). Challenging traditional insulin injection practices. *American Journal of Nursing, 99*(2), 72–74.

Haddad, A. (2001). Ethics in action. *RN, 64*(9), 25–28.

Jech, A. (2001). The next step in preventing med errors. *RN, 64*(4), 46–49.

Johanson, L. (2001). Complacency can kill. *RN, 64*(8), 49–50.

Karch, A., & Karch, F. (2001). Let the user beware. *American Journal of Nursing, 101*(2), 25.

Karch, A., & Karch, F. (2001). Take part in the solution: How to report medication errors. *American Journal of Nursing, 101*(10), 25.

Katsma, D., & Katsma, R. (2000). The myth of the 90°-angle intramuscular injection. *Nurse Educator, 25*(1), 34–37.

Koschel, M. (2001). Question of practice: Filter needles. *American Journal of Nursing, 101*(1), 75.

Kuhn, M. (1998). *Pharmacotherapeutics: a nursing process approach* (4th ed.). Philadelphia: F. A. Davis.

McConnell, E. (2001). Clinical do's & don'ts: Instilling eyedrops. *Nursing, 31*(9), 17.

McKenry, L., & Salerno, E. (2002). *Pharmacology in nursing* (21st ed.). St. Louis: C. V. Mosby.

Morris, M. (2002). When a phone order differs from the written one. *RN, 65*(1), 71.

Nicoll, L., & Hesby, A. (2002). Intramuscular injection: An integrative research review and guideline for evidence-based practice. *Applied Nursing Research, 16*(2), 149–162.

North American Nursing Diagnosis Association. (2002). *Nursing diagnoses: definitions and classification 2002–2003.* Philadelphia: Author.

Pope, B. (2002). How to administer subcutaneous and intramuscular. *Nursing, 32*(1), 50–51.

Trooskin, S. (2002). Low-technology, cost-efficient strategies for reducing medication errors. *American Journal of Infection Control, 30*(6), 351–354.

Wentz, J., Karch, A., & Karch, F. (2000). You've caught the error, now how do you fix it? *American Journal of Nursing, 100*(9), 24.

Winland-Brown, J., & Valiante, J. (2000). Effectiveness of different medication management approaches on elders' medication adherence. *Outcomes Management for Nursing Practice, 4*(4), 172–176.

Wolf, Z., Serembus, J., & Beitz, J. (2001). Clinical inference of nursing students concerning harmful outcomes after medication errors. *Nurse Educator, 26*(6), 268–270.